Both Sides of the White Coat

An Insider's Perspectives on the Critically Ill Child

Scott E. Eveloff, MD

iUniverse.com, Inc.

San Jose New York Lincoln Shanghai

Both Sides of the White Coat
An Insider's Perspectives on the Critically Ill Child

Published by People With Disabilities Press,
an imprint of iUniverse.com, inc.

For information address:
iUniverse.com, Inc.
5220 S 16th, Ste. 200
Lincoln, NE 68512
www.iuniverse.com

ISBN: 0-595-13307-X

Acknowledgements

Andrew Michael Eveloff was born on November 16, 1992. At the time of this writing Andrew is seven years old, and carries the diagnosis of congenital muscular dystrophy. Andrew's pregnancy was totally uneventful— or as uneventful as a pregnancy could be when shared by two slightly neurotic parents. The neurosis factor was elevated immeasurably because both parents also happened to be doctors. His mother was a pediatrician; and I, his father, was a pulmonologist and critical care physician—a somewhat ironic combination for a newborn child destined to have severe breathing difficulties and a life-threatening neuromuscular disease.

Problems arose soon after Andrew was born. We were allowed only a brief five or ten minutes of happiness before we realized life wasn't going exactly as expected. We had to cram a lifetime's worth of hopes and dreams for a normal baby into the five or ten minutes we had with Andrew before we realized something was wrong. Our dreams were all ripped away by the sudden, brutal reality of Andrew's severe weakness. He was immediately admitted into the Neonatal Intensive Care Unit of a hospital in Providence, Rhode Island, the beginning of our long journey.

Because we were both doctors and the parents of two other healthy children, aged six and four, we thought we were well informed. We thought we were prepared to handle most issues that would confront the most recent addition to our family. The next several days, then months, then years, would prove us to be terribly overconfident as we tried to cope with a child who was first critically ill, then terminally ill, then chronically disabled. Our personal experiences, against the background of our medical professions, gave us perspectives that we felt would apply to and, we hope, help other parents and families who find themselves in similar circumstances.

Table of Contents

Chapter 1

The Intensive Care Unit

I returned to the hospital the morning after Andrew was born, on November 17, 1992, and found myself immersed in the best and worst of medical science. Andrew had been scanned from head to toe: a kidney ultrasound, a computed tomography scan of the head, another ultrasound of his heart, multiple chest X-ray films. Known as the "shotgun approach," this deluge of tests expended health care dollars at an amazing clip and violated the rational stepwise diagnostic thinking that every medical student is cautioned to follow. It was reserved for patients who were either too sick or whose cases were too complicated to permit a more organized, step-by-step work-up. I had diligently ordered such a barrage of tests on my own patients. Now my own son was one of those very sick, and very complicated, patients.

A narrow tube had been passed through Andrew's nose into his stomach and another thin catheter had to be repetitively inserted to suction his mouth and throat, or he would have drowned in his own saliva. It was all eerily familiar, except the equipment, which was designed to be used with children, looked as if it had been made for Barbie dolls.

Out of this chaos came Dr. R, who was introduced as the attending neonatologist in charge of the Special Care Nursery. Neonatologists are specialists in charge of premature babies and newborns requiring medical care; their patients can often fit into a pair of outstretched hands. Dr. R was a diminutive physician from India who instantly put me at ease. He explained that Andrew was still having problems with his secretions, but so far, no evidence of brain or heart damage was apparent. Everyone was still confused about what had actually happened, but the neurologist was examining Andrew.

Dr. R was doing his compassionate best, but two of the worst things a doctor can hear are that "your child has a confusing illness" and that "a neurologist is examining your baby." Neurology, the study of the nervous system, is a field of medicine that covers many interesting diseases, most of which are debilitating, crippling, and completely untreatable. I did not like the sound of this. In the world of medicine, you don't want to have a confusing illness. It implies you may become a Great Case, which is a fantastically rare or illustrative disease that most doctors would like to ponder over, study, and learn from—but a disease that they would not like to become personally afflicted with themselves. From the point of view of the patient, a Great Case usually means something bad, disfiguring, or difficult to treat. Knowing I'd recently become the father of potential Great Case filled me with misery and desperation.

My wife Ruth and I didn't get much sleep that night. I went down intermittently to Special Care Nursery and walked past rows and rows of critically ill premature babies, past tiny newborns sprouting catheters and monitors out of every orifice available, to my own little son in the back of the unit. Every time I'd venture into the Special Care Nursery, I'd imagine turning the corner and seeing a crowd of doctors and nurses gathered around my son's incubator, frantically trying to revive him, shouting orders for "stat" everything.

Each time, however, I was greeted only by Andrew's calm and reassuring nurse and by Andrew himself. It started to anger me that his nurse always waited until I arrived to insert the suction catheter down his delicate little nose, noisily slurping up the saliva and mucus, until she told me it had to be done every five to ten minutes no matter who was visiting. My baby was too weak to cough or even to swallow.

Ruth and I could tolerate staying by his incubator for only a short time each visit before fleeing for the refuge of Ruth's room. There is no greater feeling of helplessness than for parents to stand within a foot of their precious newborn baby and be able to do nothing but watch, unable to help. We watched as yet another catheter was inserted into Andrew's tender little nose or mouth. We watched as another needle pricked the tiny heel for more blood to test.

We had never sunk so low as we did that day and night. The next morning, I again managed to overcome overwhelming dread and walked toward Andrew's incubator. This time, Dr. R strode up with an actual smile on his face.

"Good news, my friend," he began, holding my hands if he were a comforting man of the cloth instead of a respected academic physician and scientist. "Andrew's blood tests showed elevated muscle and liver enzymes. He may have had some perinatal asphyxia during birth that injured his muscles and spinal cord."

In everyday English, Dr. R was telling me that Andrew's problems may have been the result of a temporary loss of oxygen to his muscles and nerves, producing his terrible floppiness. It could therefore be reversible, instead of being some progressive and hopeless disease. And we were even luckier, because it appeared as if his brain had been spared! My tears were now ones of joy. Dr. R followed us as we rushed over to Andrew's incubator to see him. Dr. R kept up a constant stream of good news.

"Andrew is one of the most alert babies I've seen in here, another very good sign his brain is all right. We've got to stay very hopeful." Then he actually came up and hugged each of us. I felt as if a huge weight had been lifted from me. We stayed with Andrew for quite a while after that. I really looked at Andrew's blue eyes for the first time; they were indeed looking around intently at his surroundings. Not even the constant stream of saliva from his mouth could dampen the new surge of hope we felt. We could almost ignore the intravenous catheter poking into Andrew's scalp, the feeding tube in his nose, the puncture marks on each heel, the beeping of his oxygen monitor, the painful repetitive suctioning…almost. It truly is amazing what people suffering through the intensive care unit (ICU) become used to—or become thankful for.

That night I dared to make a few optimistic phone calls to family with the good news—"good" in that our child had only suffered possible asphyxia, or injury from low oxygen, instead of having something really bad. Like I said, it's amazing what families dealing with critical illness become thankful for. For most parents, asphyxia usually means brain damage, eventual cerebral palsy, and disheartening impairment. For doctors, asphyxia invokes images of costly malpractice lawsuits. To us, as doctors and as parents, asphyxia actually meant that Andrew could possibly heal; his condition could even resolve.

But the roller coaster had only just begun. Upon entering the Special Care Nursery the next morning, Ruth and I were met by a physician who specialized in newborn babies, called neonates. Her academic title was "Neonatology Fellow," which meant she was training in the highly specialized field involving critically ill newborns (a fellow is a trainee in any medical sub-specialty beyond basic medical training in more generalized areas such as internal medicine or pediatrics). She told us that Andrew's secretions weren't getting any better. In fact, to protect Andrew from drowning in his secretions, the fellow was recommending intubation for airway protection. For me, this was the final irony. Her words hit me like a slap in the face. How many times had I informed patients and families that we needed to put a special tube down the major breathing airway, so secretions and saliva from the mouth would not drip into the lungs and cause pneumonia? I always recommended intubation in a calm, dispassionate manner, as a mechanic might recommend the need for a new transmission if a major leak were spotted. Now I was on the other side of the fence, listening as the fellow's dispassionate voice recommended something I knew to be very serious indeed.

The fact is, either as a child or as an adult, you have to be in very bad shape to be unable to protect your airway. It's one of the most basic reflexes humans have. Anyone who has ever coughed and sputtered after only a small amount of water went down the wrong way knows how the human body values a clean, dry airway and works to protect it. Only disastrous events leave the airway vulnerable, such as strokes, severe intoxication, or paralysis. But for my newborn son? It was unthinkable.

Immediately upon hearing the fellow's words, images of my son with his throat violated by a tube blinded me. I projected Andrew years into the future, picturing him languishing in a nursing home for babies until he was old enough to graduate to a real adult nursing home. Dr. R solemnly seconded the need for airway protection. And suddenly Ruth and I were again engulfed in despair and anguish.

We came back after the tube had been placed. It was much smaller than the tubes I was used to; it almost resembled a straw. I didn't want to admit it, but Andrew actually looked more comfortable, and he was at last able to sleep without constantly fighting for breath. I hated to admit that the intubation was for the best, because with each new intervention, my son came to resemble the older, sicker, dying patients I took care of daily.

I dreaded the morning visit to the Special Care Nursery the following day, but we were met with better news this time. Dr. R put his arm around Ruth and me and told us that Andrew had had a comfortable night, his urine output was back to normal, and some movement was coming back. Andrew's grip seemed much stronger. Dr. R kept repeating his very good feeling about "your little Andrew." And just like that, we were sure this all had happened to make sure we'd never take anything for granted, and of course it was going to work out just fine.

Andrew himself truly did appear more robust, if such a term could be used to describe an infant covered more by monitors and bandages than by soft skin. His eyes were always darting back and forth. His movements seemed more vigorous. He'd gone without food since birth, and now Dr. R and his fellows wanted to start feeding him through his veins and possibly start him on breast milk if all went well.

Then the final magic moment of that morning came: we were allowed to hold him for the first time. It was far removed from those Nescafe moments on television, where parent and perfect baby tenderly bond just before a good cup of coffee. We had to balance three different monitor wires, the endotracheal tube, and a baby as floppy as any Raggedy Ann doll ever made. But it still felt wonderful. And we'd had our fill of coffee.

Unfortunately, Dr. R's consistently optimistic message was gradually causing us to feel deep feelings of resentment toward any other health care professional who dared voice more pessimistic views of Andrew's condition. Now that Dr. R's unflagging belief in Andrew's certain recovery had been validated, at least temporarily, we were coming to see the neurologist, the pediatrician, and some of the hospital's fellows as the enemies. They were doctors who couldn't see past their cold, scientific training enough to admit their initial impressions had been wrong. We were shooting the messengers—as long as they were the messengers of any news or opinions about our son we chose not to believe.

The depth of our denial was actually much more profound than we realized at the time. In fact, Ruth and I considered ourselves ahead of the game in terms of insight and acceptance of our son's situation. After all, we were doctors, Ruth a pediatrician, which obviously endowed us with powers over the standard parent in the same situation.

The lessons born out of these experiences have shaped my professional and personal life and have remained vivid in my life years later. Professionally, I accept that doctors may have to bear the brunt of news too horrible for most people to even comprehend. It stands me in good stead when faced with irate, angry, or irrational families of critically ill or terminally ill patients. Absorbing their pain, even as a well-intentioned or blameless scapegoat, still causes me or any other doctor far less pain than the anguish such people have to face daily. If such a role becomes one more unwritten responsibility of a physician, then so be it.

From a patient's perspective, it certainly is easier to appreciate and reward bearers of good news about a loved one who is sick. It is harder to accept that bad news and more pessimistic opinions, especially when delivered compassionately, may be closer to reality and may deserve as much, if not greater, appreciation.

Personally, I've remained more aware that the superior knowledge and experience I have obtained from hospitals, other doctors, and disease processes may only create a false sense of security when faced with personal tragedy and illness. Beyond the most basic illnesses, the human body and its responses are simply too complex and unpredictable for anyone to fully comprehend and predict the course of severe illness, whether they're supported by a medical degree or not. This knowledge was and continues to be very humbling, which is not altogether so bad.

Unfortunately, living within the surreal world of coping with a critically ill child left little room for self-realization or growth. Even as we were still enjoying our new sense of hope, the ICU roller coaster continued to take us on a dizzying ride of highs and lows. Dr. R had recommended that special X-ray films be taken of Andrew's brain and spinal cord just to make sure there had been no injury. Flush with optimism and confidence, we agreed. It was only precautionary, and Andrew was going to get better anyway, right?

Things didn't go smoothly. They had so much trouble sedating Andrew for the scan that the doctors decided to artificially paralyze him with drugs in order to keep him perfectly still. The breathing tube still in his lungs allowed machines to breathe for him while he was paralyzed. I found the need to administer paralyzing drugs upsetting. I am particularly sensitive about paralyzing drugs, since they are used fairly often in the adult ICU. These drugs are actually related to the drug curare, which is known to many as the drug South American natives tipped their arrows with to kill animals and enemies alike. Paralyzing drugs are also among the last drugs administered to convicts during their execution by lethal injection. Curare and its modern derivatives temporarily poison nerve endings and create total paralysis. Patients can't move or blink, and they can't even breathe on their own. Doctors therefore rely on a breathing machine hooked up to a tube, like the kind Andrew had. Patients can't move, but they remain perfectly awake and alert unless also sedated, and they remain able to feel and sense pain, since the drugs don't affect the nerves controlling sensation. I had seen firsthand what happens when patients aren't properly sedated before being paralyzed; at least for adults it is terrifying to be suddenly unable to move but yet remain totally aware. It seemed the greatest of medical ironies to paralyze a child who was just recovering from severe weakness.

But now my baby was paralyzed and totally dependent on a breathing machine for his very life—different only by virtue of age and size from the suffering victims of tragic illnesses that I paralyze and breathe for in my own ICU in the name of medical treatment. His tiny body and innocent face made the situation all the more obscene. The roller coaster had again plunged down into a deep trough of panic and despair as I sat and watched my motionless child. I was now sure he would never be able to breathe on his own; vivid images of the tracheostomy tube again intruded into my thoughts.

The next day, however, once again brought an unexpected change, this time for the better. I was hanging onto the roller coaster for dear life. Andrew had actually been weaned off the breathing machine once the drugs had worn off, and he had done so well that they had taken the tube out totally! This time I couldn't stop the tears. The constant upheavals and the pounding our emotions had taken with each day's reversal of fortune had left Ruth and me unable to assimilate any new change, whether for better or for worse.

But "better" came. Over the course of the week, Andrew steadily improved. His oxygen level was staying up, his secretions were no longer drowning him, and of course Dr. R stood by his conviction of eventual total recovery. They had even started feeding him breast milk through the tube in his stomach. Once again, we dared to believe everything would work out for the best. After all, hadn't we been through more hell in one week than we deserved to go through in a lifetime?

The weekend saw nothing but more improvement. Andrew remained very alert, and his grip seemed stronger and stronger. Each time we were allowed to hold him, it was accomplished with fewer and fewer devices getting in the way. Dr. R had become downright bubbly when he greeted us in the mornings. What would we have done without him? It is difficult to believe that two previously assured physicians would place themselves so entirely into the hands of another doctor, an equal, and feel so helpless without him. Is that what patients, or the parents of patients, feel under such conditions? Over the years, with more experiences as a physician and as a parent, I believe that patients feel even more dependent on a doctor they trust. I have remained aware since then of the power that members of my profession wield and have tried to live up to such expectations.

Andrew celebrated his first week of life still in the Special Care Nursery, but was almost off oxygen and most of his monitors. The only decision left was how far to go to rule out any other neurologic disease besides simple injury from some hidden birth trauma. It was virtually unanimous that he was doing too well to rock the boat, and the hospital pathologist felt any biopsy would be difficult to interpret anyway. The way was cleared for us to take our miracle baby home.

We said our good-byes to the multitude of nurses, doctors, and other staff members, then strolled out the door with Andrew. I reflected to myself, overconfidently, how maybe some good had come out of that week's roller coaster ride through the other side of medicine. Not many doctors have had the experience of suffering so immediately with their patients. I walked out of the hospital with a new baby, a new appreciation of life, and a new insight into the lives of the people I served daily. I felt almost like I was waking up out of a bad dream: I felt terror, but I also felt immeasurable relief at being able to return to normal life after awakening. As we carried Andrew into the house for the first time, everything was exactly the same as it had been. The crib and changing table were set up and decorated, the bottles and nipples were washed and ready, and musical mobiles were hanging up. Everything seemed so normal that it was easy to believe that the trial of the last week had never really happened.

We settled into the newborn routine surprisingly easily. Andrew took to breast-feeding. He cried, smiled, and pooped, and he depended on us for everything, just like any other new baby. His limpness only served to accentuate normal newborn helplessness and endeared him all the more to us.

There were some differences, however. We made sure he was exposed to as few germs as possible. For two doctors, this meant rather draconian measures were enacted. Our other two children wore surgical masks all the time, since one or the other usually had a cold. My parents were forced to wear masks around Andrew as well. Between the incessant hand-washing and surgical masks, it probably seemed to any visitor that we were always just about ready to operate on Andrew instead of preparing change his diapers. Our excesses would have made for a great sitcom sketch, I'm sure.

Andrew's two weeks in the hospital and one week at home had aged me much beyond a simple three weeks. I was confident, however, that our increasingly normal routine would quickly prove restorative. Toward the end of that first week home, Andrew developed mild nasal congestion and had a little more trouble breast-feeding. Soon after that, Dr. R stopped by to say hello and make sure we were doing all right—an emotional well-being house call, as it were; it was something else I have taken to heart over the years. He looked at Andrew, held his little hand just as he had done in the Special Care Nursery, and declared him as having nothing more than a little cold. Dr. R felt Andrew would certainly bounce back again, as he had done previously.

Armed with such reassurance, we took Andrew's congestion in stride and dutifully tried to get him to feed. The nights became a little more difficult, however. He would only sleep for a short time before waking up crying. Each time we would shove a bottle in his mouth, then a pacifier. Next, we would rock him, and finally we'd lay him in his crib until he cried himself to sleep. It remained so easy to believe that this was just normal, irritating newborn behavior, because our baby *was* normal—back from the dead and responsible for several hundred thousand dollars' worth of hospital bills, but normal.

We finally called Andrew's pediatrician when we could no longer deny that something was not quite right. In the pediatrician's examining room, I had the opportunity to take a really good look at our baby, lying on a stark table under the bright glare of an unforgiving overhead light.

Andrew appeared weak, frail, almost pasty. In fact, he looked downright sickly. It looked as if we hadn't fed him for over a week. When had this happened? He had been so healthy after leaving the hospital—hadn't he? Had we really wished our baby to be normal so much that we had totally overlooked his inability to suck, his weight loss, his progressive difficulty breathing? We obviously had, we two intelligent doctor-parents, because Andrew's pediatrician took one look and listen and recommended we take Andrew to the emergency room immediately.

Gazing at Andrew, I realized the pediatrician wasn't being unreasonable or overly pessimistic at all. For the first time in over a week, I felt my eyes grow hot with tears. And worse, that sick feeling in my stomach was back. It couldn't be happening again. We'd had our share already. I tried asking questions as we bundled Andrew up in his snowsuit, but my voice couldn't stop quivering. We didn't know it then, but the only time we would be a happy, unconcerned, and "normal" family of five ended with that visit to the pediatrician. We had packed a lifetime of family bliss into a single week.

Andrew's congestion was destined to become much more than just a cold. Andrew was destined to stay in an ICU, graduating to one for older children instead of for newborns. A bad combination of continued respiratory muscle weakness and the miserably unfortunate coincidence of catching a viral infection led to worsening breathing difficulty. The pediatrician was right: Andrew needed immediate help. We left for the hospital immediately. After I dropped Ruth and Andrew off at the emergency room, I parked the car and returned to find them ensconced in one of the cubicles. Andrew had once again been subjected to poking and prodding; again, he had been punctured with needles to draw blood samples. He wore a tiny oxygen mask, and he had just been X-rayed. I was told that his breathing had improved after receiving a respiratory treatment. Once again, I was on the other side of terrifyingly familiar ground, watching someone with all the familiar breathing problems getting all the familiar, almost routine, treatments, X-ray films, and tests. The gasping asthmatic, however, was my son this time.

The real shock came when we were told Andrew was being admitted to the Pediatric ICU. First he had been in the Neonatal Intensive Care Unit (NICU); now he needed to visit the Pediatric Intensive Care Unit (PICU). As we sat around in Andrew's newest home, a much older, dilapidated unit with withered children obscured by oxygen tents, we felt incredibly out of place. We were too knowledgeable about our son's illness and the medical treatments it required to wander in bewildered numbness around the unit, but we had too much at stake on a personal level to deal with everything rationally. It was in this frame of mind that we took in the first piece of definite news from one of the residents staffing the PICU that night. She informed us that the swabs taken from Andrew's nose and throat had come back positive for RSV, or respiratory syncytial virus. It is a virus common in the winter months among infants and children and is very contagious. It can lead to wheezing, pneumonia, and death, even if the affected child didn't already have a severe problem to begin with.

Things only worsened the next day. His breathing became faster as he struggled to breathe against worsening congestion. More ominous to us, his physician-parents, however, were the repeated arterial blood gas measurements taken from him. An arterial blood gas is a sample of blood obtained directly from an artery. It is quite a bit more painful than the standard blood draw, which is taken from a less sensitive vein, and may require agonizing probing by the needle before the actual artery is punctured. Seeing Andrew suffer each arterial stick was painful enough, but it paled in comparison with the test's findings. Andrew's carbon dioxide level was steadily rising, which meant he was becoming unable to breathe out the carbon dioxide his body manufactured. (Carbon dioxide is a toxic by-product of the human metabolism; oxygen is the good, beneficial air breathed in, and carbon dioxide is exhaled). It meant Andrew was tiring in his struggle to breathe. If he continued to lose the battle, he would have to be put on a respirator, with a breathing tube once again violating his throat.

And once again, I was faced with watching my son endure what I decided for my patients in the adult ICU. I knew the discomfort, the implications, of putting someone on life support, which that breathing tube and the ventilator represented. Many patients recovered from such dire straits and were eventually weaned off the ventilator. Unfortunately, I knew too much about what the patients went through before recovering, and I knew too much about the people who didn't recover once this desperate point had been reached. Only much later did it occur to me that some of the patients and families to whom I had impatiently explained why such drastic measures had become necessary had maybe felt the same panic and sense of finality that I was feeling now.

Andrew's doctors decided to tough it out with Andrew and tried to avoid putting him on a breathing machine as long as possible. It meant more arterial blood gas assessments, careful observation, and unrelenting agony for Ruth and me as we awaited those telling numbers. As if to further underscore the gravity of the situation, Andrew was started on a special inhaled version of a drug to treat RSV. It was clear now that he had developed an actual pneumonia from the RSV. The inhaled drug is called ribavirin, and it had to be administered inside a special plastic tent that kept the patient isolated from everyone else. The patient is draped in plastic and the ribavirin administered under the plastic into the air the patient breathes.

For the next three days, Andrew was surrounded by two layers of thick plastic. He was totally cut off from human touch or voice, caressed only by an occasional gloved hand sneaked between sheets of plastic; he was warmed only by humidified oxygen and ribavirin vapors. It was a disheartening feeling, knowing Andrew was immersed in the fumes of the same medicine that all his health care providers took extraordinary precautions to avoid because of its toxicity. My emptiness was matched only by the anxiety of wondering when in those endless first three days Andrew would succumb to the virus the ribavirin attempted to control and by my helplessness at being unable to assist or even provide a gentle caress of love as he struggled to breathe.

Whether it was the ribavirin, Andrew's strength, or other, more intangible, forces, our son began turning the corner. After hovering on the verge of losing the fight to breathe on his own and clear his own secretions, his carbon dioxide levels began improving, and his breathing became less rapid and difficult. The ribavirin was pronounced a success and finally stopped. When the nurses started unwrapping the plastic tenting from around his bed, it seemed more to me that they were unwrapping a special gift for us. It was quite possibly the best present I could ever remember unwrapping.

For the second time, we had to get used to holding him as much as we wanted. His oxygen was weaned down, then off, and he even started to eat a little more, although he remained pitifully thin. The entire family once again started to breathe a little easier, one more literally than others. We actually dared to contemplate the future again, a future, we hoped, without any more ICUs in it.

The Experience of the ICU

For adults sick enough to be hospitalized in an ICU, and for their concerned relatives and friends, the experience can be one of the most intimidating they will ever face. For parents and friends of a child or infant requiring care in a NICU or PICU, the confusion and anxiety are infinitely magnified. For those unfortunate children themselves, the ICU must be the stuff of nightmares.

Imagine it: complex machines at each bedside, some continuously moving, hissing, or buzzing. Others flash bright neon or green patterns of heart rates, blood pressure, oxygen levels, and many other vital secrets for anyone to see. Intravenous fluids on poles with two or three infusions going at once spring up like strange, futuristic trees. All these intimidating devices reach out their tentacles of tubes, catheters, and pumps to surround and overwhelm the patient at their center.

Then there are the inhabitants of the PICU. They usually travel in packs on their daily rounds—the attending physician confidently leading; overtired residents following, just having come off a sleepless night on call; impatient residents, just starting their tour of duty, trying to push ahead; and medical students bringing up the rear, eager to shamelessly goggle at the next interesting case. For the sickest of patients, the doctors come wrapped in gowns, masks, and gloves. They surround each bed and its tiny patient, peer, prod, examine some more, pronounce unintelligible words that must somehow be very important, and then move on to the next bed or room. At odd times during the rest of the day, other staff members scurry in, adjust a ventilator or an infusion, acknowledge parents and children with a brief nod and a slightly embarrassed smile, and then scurry out.

It could all just as easily be the set for a movie about a mad doctor, full of mysterious experiments and devices that create an atmosphere of suspicion and fear. Is this an unfair exaggeration of what happens when children or babies require critical care? Great strides have been made to create more nurturing environments, and pediatric units are especially sensitive to the emotions and anxieties of children and parents. Nonetheless, the reality is that the ICU is the place with the concentration of the sickest of the sick, where technology outstrips the imaginations of most laypeople, where the life and death of patients can literally be played out on a minute-to-minute basis, whether those patients are 90 hours old or 90 years old.

Definitions

An ICU can mean different things under different conditions. In smaller hospitals, the ICU may handle cases that simply require closer nursing observation or better monitoring. In larger hospitals and in most university hospitals, the ICU caters to the very sickest patients, many of whom are almost at the point of death upon their arrival to the unit or shortly thereafter.

The NICU is for newborn patients only. It handles newborns who develop a wide range of problems immediately before or after birth. Premature birth, sick or diabetic mothers, maternal or newborn fever, and respiratory problems at birth may all land a newborn in the NICU. Because newborn babies are extremely fragile and very susceptible to infection even when they are healthy, it doesn't take much to recommend their placement in such a setting. Sometimes just being the product of a twin or triplet birth may require a short stay in the NICU. Having a baby stay there is not automatically a cause for panic. But neonates in the NICU may be at the far other end of the spectrum as well, requiring emergent full life support for heart and lung failure, low blood pressure, or overwhelming infection. Most people never actually hear of the NICU. In the same spirit that drives pediatricians to attach cute little warm and fuzzy teddy bears to their stethoscopes, these units are more commonly called by kinder and gentler names, such as "Special Care Nursery," to name one example. In contrast, an adult medical ICU *is* the ICU; it is not given a code name such as the Focused Revival and Treatment Unit, for example. There is certainly something to be said for a specialty that at least makes an effort at to be warm and fuzzy under such trying conditions, to be sure.

The PICU is a step closer to an adult ICU. Infants who have left the hospital after birth and older children are hospitalized in the PICU when they become severely ill. Newborns who have gone home with their parents do not return to the NICU if they get sick again because they presumably have been exposed to outside viruses and bacteria (the infamous *germs* that people always refer to) that could spread rapidly among the other neonates. Older children in the PICU can be quite sick, suffering from severe infections or breathing problems, head injuries, coma from near-drowning or other childhood accidents, or postoperative complications.

Both the NICU and the PICU are for exactly that: intensive care. One-on-one nursing care is the rule, as is constant monitoring of all vital life functions. Many types of health care support staff interact to deliver specialized services around the clock: respiratory therapists deliver inhaled medicines and chest physical therapy; dietitians supervise feeding by either intravenous catheters or feeding tubes (such as those Andrew required); radiology technicians go from patient to patient, shooting black-and-white snapshots; physical and occupational therapists caress, stretch, and lift; and the list could go on. There are many complaints that patients and families voice when in the ICU, but physical loneliness is rarely one of them.

Technology in the ICU: Monitors and Ventilators

The most striking aspect of the ICU is probably the overwhelming array of machines and technology that surrounds each patient. When that patient is an infant, the machinery attending to them can swallow them up. Babies can be enclosed within layers of beeping, clicking metal and plastic catheters, tubing, and hanging wires. It may start to resemble a weird jungle of technology separating parents from their children. Newborns, or any child, for that matter, deserve to be surrounded by stuffed animals and bright pillows, with happy mobiles hanging overhead instead of plastic tubing. The ICU environment will rarely be anything other than brutal for parents, but understanding these machines may make it a little less intimidating.

The ICU's monitor may appear easy to understand and usually draws the attention of most parents first. The monitor is the screen above the patient that displays continuous tracings of heart rate, blood pressure, temperature, oxygen level, and specialized internal readings, when available. Even if parents tried, it would be difficult to ignore these numbers because of the machine's beeping and because of the riveting neon colors of the tracings.

Numbers are easy to understand and focus on, and ICU monitors display them for anyone to see. Agonized parents commonly sit endlessly at the bedside. I know Ruth and I felt we had to be there, unable to physically help or intervene but feeling as if just our presence could somehow be sensed by Andrew and make a difference. But with so little to do, and prohibited from even holding their babies, parents almost inevitably turn attention to that neon billboard of numbers and tracings.

Because of this, some parents and other relatives become unwitting surrogate bedside physicians. Many become fixated on heart rates going up. The percentage of oxygen in the blood (actually, the percentage of a hemoglobin molecule that is saturated with oxygen. Hemoglobin is the substance in red blood cells that is responsible for carrying oxygen) is another favorite value to focus on, especially as oxygen level equals life to many people. Parents often feel the need to alert ICU staff to fluctuations in the numbers or to question why doctors permit certain values to persist. Although done out of the best of intentions, this behavior can be detrimental to the already fragile network of relatives and professionals supporting each patient.

Certain guidelines may help with this situation. The ICU is crawling with health care providers. When they are not physically at the bedside, they still have access to the information on the monitor via centralized screens. Vital information is always accessible to appropriate staff members, making parents' constant updates unnecessary. Fluctuations occur routinely in many body functions and usually require no specific intervention. As many monitoring systems have programmed low thresholds to help troubleshooting, routine fluctuations may set off alarms but may still not require attention. Most important of all, the one thing there *is* a shortage of in the ICU is simple tenderness. Gentle caressing of a child, offering reassuring words, giving a hug if catheters and tubing permit, and reading a story all contribute as much, if not more, to a child's well-being than all the machines and medicines. Fixating only on electrical tracings and oxygen fluctuations may take away from the intangible support that only parents or siblings can offer. Parents really need to be care providers first, not health care providers.

The monitor may be the most obvious piece of equipment to study while whiling away the hours in the ICU. But the ventilator is central to intensive care therapy of critically ill infants and children who can't breathe on their own. In premature newborns whose lungs have not had enough time to mature, the ventilator plays an especially crucial role. Many different types of ventilators exist, providing a multitude of different ways to give breath to a patient. Nonetheless, this complicated machine does not have to be so intimidating. Ventilators are machines that essentially push oxygen-enriched air in and out of the lungs through a plastic tube inserted through the mouth or nose, down between the vocal cords, and into the largest airway of the lungs. The air may be vibrated into the lungs with many tiny breaths or delivered under higher pressure with larger breaths. The breaths themselves are made up of varying amounts of oxygen, sometimes mixed in with special inhaled medications for premature babies. But ventilators are really just complicated bellows, forcing air in and out of the lungs.

Ventilators should not be confused with oxygen masks or with the nasal prongs placed under patients' noses. This misconception is understandable; almost every soap opera or TV show portrays critically ill patients whose only source of medical support, despite suffering overwhelming trauma, is that little oxygen tubing running into their noses. These devices are great for allowing the actor to give melodramatic speeches, but they are lousy for really keeping such patients alive. Prongs and simple masks provide additional oxygen to patients who can still breathe on their own. The much more complicated ventilator takes over breathing for the patient and delivers much higher levels of oxygen through a tube that is actually inserted into the internal airway instead of through simple tubing running into the nose or a through a mask resting on a patient's face.

Ventilators can be extremely nerve-wracking because they are almost always beeping, buzzing, or lighting up. Most ventilators have low threshold for sounding an alarm, and those annoying buzzes will signal a life-threatening event. They must sound loudly, however, because they are actually keeping the patient alive, and any real interruption in that function needs to be recognized immediately. Ventilators are the ultimate life-support, or life-sustaining, machine in the ICU.

Feeding the Patient in the ICU

Even something as basic as nutrition takes on added complexity in critically ill children and infants. As an interested observer of other families in the Special Care Nursery and then in the PICU, I saw many parents, mothers in particular, fixate on the need to start bottle-feeding their babies as early as possible—even babies on maximal ventilator support, too fragile to even be lifted out of the incubator. They often become frustrated, even angry, when doctors deemed alternative means of feeding their children necessary or when breast milk supplementation had to be delayed. Moreover, those bags of clear intravenous fluid constantly infusing into a child's veins do not give nutrition and are not substitutes for food. Even if these infusions are mixed with dextrose (a form of sugar), adequate nutrition is not provided.

Newborns, children, and adults on ventilators, with breathing tubes in their mouths going into the lungs, cannot suck or chew on anything. Even after being removed from the ventilator and having the tube taken out of their (2) mouths, many infants are simply too weak, and have to work too hard just to breathe, to take adequate nutrition on their own in the normal way. Newborns sick enough to be in the ICU need all the rest they can get during this period of severe illness. It may seem hard to believe, but even trying to suck on an offered nipple may tire the infant and delay recovery.

There are certainly times for starting natural feeding, ideally with breast milk, but there are also times when this natural approach is inappropriate. Other means of giving calories and nutrition to one's child may become necessary. Bonding, breast-feeding, and natural feeding may unfortunately, of necessity, be superseded by the need to more effectively support a weakened infant.

It should also be emphasized that during severe illness, the human body may burn up calories at a tremendous rate, even though outwardly an infant may appear to be lying quietly amidst tubing and catheters. Infants and children do not even have to have a fever to burn up this tremendous amount of calories. So even if they have recovered enough to suck on a bottle or chew and eat on their own (as in older children), supplemental feeding may still be necessary to meet their increased caloric requirements. In these situations, the doctor does not irrationally delay maternal nurturing; he or she may be acknowledging that the child requires extra nutrition to make up for the nutritional losses suffered while in the PICU.

If supplemental feeding is deemed necessary, tube feeding is the best choice. A small, flexible tube is placed through the infant's nose directly into the stomach, and liquid feedings are then infused. The tube itself may appear intrusive and uncomfortable, but most of the discomfort takes place during its insertion. Once in, the tube itself causes little pain. Unlike the breathing tube, a prolonged period with such a feeding tube in place does not prevent attempts to allow natural sucking or feeding. The breathing tube invades the vocal cords and airway, places where solid objects are never supposed to go, and is thus much more irritating and uncomfortable. The feeding tube is placed where food and liquids routinely go: into the esophagus, and nowhere near the vocal cords and lungs.

Unfortunately, and all too commonly, the stomach and intestines do not work in critically ill patients. In these situations, the infusion of complex nutrients in intravenous fluid can be dripped through a large vein.

Supplying a patient with all nutritional needs through a vein instead of the natural way, through the gut, is called total parenteral nutrition, or TPN. This differs substantially from the routine intravenous fluids which I've already explained cannot be used for nutrition. TPN usually has to be infused through a sterile catheter placed in a large, deep vein in the neck or upper chest. In contrast, standard hydrating fluids need only a small intravenous catheter in any small superficial arm or leg vein.

The complexity of administering TPN only starts with placing an appropriate catheter in a deep central vein. Bleeding, lung puncture, or accidental puncturing of an unintended vessel may occur when the catheter is placed. If not watched closely, electrolyte (blood chemistry) and blood mineral abnormalities can be generated as the complicated mixture is infused. Infections are also an increased risk with TPN because of the indwelling catheter and the glucose (sugar)- and fat-laden solution running through it.

At every step of the way, therefore, TPN is a complicated option for providing nutrition and shouldn't be taken lightly. As tempting as it may be to insist on the apparently easy alternative of "feeding my child through his veins," thus avoiding an uncomfortable feeding tube, TPN should really be reserved for infants and children who aren't able to get nutrition any other way.

Medications in the PICU

It would be impossible to adequately explain about all the medications a child could be subjected to while hospitalized in the ICU. Certain medications, however, deserve comment, either because they are used frequently or because their effects are extreme.

Among the latter group of medications are paralyzing agents, such as the medication Andrew received when he had to be perfectly still in order for an X-ray scan to be taken. These drugs literally paralyze all the body's muscles. Obviously, such medications can only be used in an ICU and under very restricted circumstances. They are used more often in adult ICUs, but they do have uses in infants and children, as demonstrated by Andrew's experience. These drugs paralyze all muscles of the body with perhaps unexpected, if not frightening, results. Eyelids can't open, facial muscles don't move, and breathing muscles don't work. It all means that these patients will die of suffocation unless a ventilator takes over breathing for them.

Why are medications with such terrifying power used at all? Certainly a parent might understandably be quite reluctant to permit his or her child to be given such medication. As in Andrew's case, however, total immobility is sometimes required for a test, and paralysis must be accomplished if the patient is too confused or too young to cooperate. Parents are informed when such drugs are required. In turn, parents need to understand that very careful consideration has probably been put into the doctor's recommendation to administer these drugs. Parents and other family members also need to be told that patients can still hear normally when they are paralyzed, although generally patients are sedated into unawareness first. Constant bedside comforting becomes even more important during these times. There really is no way to tell for certain if a paralyzed patient is awake or sedated, although sweating or rapid heart rate may be signs.

In addition to paralyzing drugs, doctors often use powerful sedating medications in the ICU. Such drugs are vitally important when a patient is paralyzed, as they allay the very real and substantial anxiety a paralyzed child or adult may feel. However, almost every intervention during hospitalization, as well as the hospitalization itself, with all the strange people and machines, can provoke anxiety in a child. Sedatives may therefore be frequently required. Effects always wear off, and mild sleepiness or grogginess is a small price to pay for ensuring a loved one's comfort.

An increasingly common medication used almost exclusively in the NICU is called *surfactant*. Many premature infants have severe problems breathing because their lungs are too underdeveloped to make adequate amounts of surfactant, which is produced by normal lungs in both children and adults. This substance essentially permits the small air sacs in the lungs to expand and fill with air. Without it, a premature newborn's lungs become airless and collapsed. Recent medical advances allow doctors to administer artificial surfactant directly into the lungs through the breathing tubes connecting the infants to their ventilators. This treatment has revolutionized the treatment of premature infants and has saved many of their lives. Parents may not even be aware it is being administered, since it is given through equipment that is probably already in place.

It is important for parents to understand that physicians will not review in detail all the medications the doctors recommend for use, including their indications and possible side effects, unless they are known to cause extreme effects, such as paralyzing agents. However, physicians and nurses should always attempt to answer parents' specific questions about medications or unlabeled intravenous fluids as forthrightly as possible. Even momentary attention to specific parental concerns about the substance being infused into their child can go a long way toward easing the anxiety that invariably affects patients and family members in the ICU. Rarely do parents insist on long, disruptive explanations. Brief, directed answers, even to technical questions posed by parents, go a long way to foster an empathic instead of adversarial atmosphere.

Sleep (or the Lack Thereof) and the ICU

Many natural body processes that fail during overwhelming illness need to be taken over by artificial means until healing occurs and function returns. Feeding tubes or TPN replace eating and drinking; ventilators take over breathing; passive stretching and physical therapy combat immobility borne by paralysis or weakness—in short, vital, basic needs can be totally taken over by technology. There is one basic need, however, that cannot be as easily replaced by technology: sleep. In fact, not only is the basic biologic function of sleep commonly disrupted by the ICU and all its workings, but sleep deficiency may be all but ignored.

Most people have experienced the fatigue, the inability to concentrate, and the irritability caused by a sleepless or interrupted night. Most of us never really appreciate how important uninterrupted sleep is until we are forced to do without it. Yet for many children, infants, and adults requiring ICU care, restorative sleep may be disturbed night after night. Even the act of breathing on ventilator maybe enough to disrupt sleep. Add to this the discomfort of being virtually tethered down by tubes, catheters, and monitors, the constant beeping of various machines or infusion pumps, the interruptions by therapists for breathing treatments or other therapies day and night, and it becomes surprising if satisfying sleep weren't lost by patients.

Moreover, in many ICUs, "morning" X-ray scans, and "morning" blood work are taken around 4:30 in the morning, so results are ready for the doctors when they start their early morning rounds. This routine is great for the medical teams, as it allows them to use their time productively, but such awakenings are the last sleep-disturbing straw for many patients who had just fallen back to sleep from previous interruptions.

Many patients, therefore, become chronically sleep-deprived while hospitalized, especially during an ICU stay. Unlike disruption of other processes, such as breathing or eating, a suitable artificial means of restoring or replacing sleep has not been found. Administration of sedatives would appear to be a reasonable solution, and in fact their use can go a long way toward reducing the impact of nocturnal awakenings. However, sedating medications can also carry over into daytime hours. In children already sleepy from the previous disturbed night, this prolonged effect may lead to even greater daytime drowsiness or actual sleep. Over time, a child's sleep–wake cycle may become first confused, then reversed. What sleep they manage to obtain comes in brief periods in both daytime and nighttime hours and tends to be less restorative.

This kind of sleep loss and sleep irregularity is frustrating to parents, children, and staff alike. However, disrupted or absolute lack of sleep can actually have a more ominous impact on recovery from critical illness. Sleep loss may cause respiratory and upper airway muscles to weaken. In children or infants whom doctors are trying to wean from a ventilator or who already have problems breathing on their own, sleep loss may be enough to tip the scales from recovery to setback. Lack of sleep can also impair the brain's ability to respond to changes in oxygen or carbon dioxide, further complicating the course of recovery of a child—especially a premature newborn—suffering from respiratory complications.

Sleep loss may also in some ways affect the immune system, which is the body's defense system against infections. This effect is not unequivocally proven, but it is supported by several laboratory studies. The immune system cannot be seen the way large organs such as the lungs, brain, or heart can be seen. The tiny molecules of antibodies and the cells that produce and work with them all circulate in the blood and cannot be seen by the naked eye. But in any case, sleep loss, unfortunately quite prevalent in the ICU, can have many ill effects on the human body and can contribute to both physical and emotional problems in this already fragile group. So can anything be done?

Most adult and pediatric ICUs have become much more aware of the problem. Many units work to consolidate sleep among critically ill patients. Reducing unnecessary tests and awakenings at night, keeping overhead lights on a regular day-night cycle, reducing conversations among staff during nighttime hours, and carefully regulating the use of sedatives all help to restore the quality and quantity of sleep. These strategies are very helpful, but I also firmly believe that allowing parents virtually unrestricted access to their babies' or children's bedsides at night is extremely important. Parents would be right at their children's side at home to comfort them back to sleep after they awoke from physical discomfort or bad dreams. Why not use such natural parental comfort in the ICU, where physical discomfort—and probably bad dreams—are so magnified?

To help their children get the sleep they need, parents should not hesitate to point out to hospital staff when interruptions for tests or monitoring could be better done during daytime hours. Sometimes medical treatment plans make perfect sense to everyone except the patients they are intended for. Patients commonly receive inhaled medicines on a regular basis to treat asthma and relieve bronchial spasms. But receiving this treatment can be disruptive. Many of my own patients have complained that they were awakened out of a sound sleep to receive such a treatment. They had been sleeping soundly up until the treatment without any breathing problems, but they felt miserable the next day because they had been unable to return to sleep after a treatment that was supposed to make them feel better.

Pointing out such well-intentioned but misguided nocturnal treatments may save everyone involved many otherwise frustrating days and nights. Parents looking out for their children's welfare should also realize, however, that bodily processes are active around the clock. Medical treatments designed to take over for these processes when something goes wrong must, of necessity, also be administered around the clock. Medical interventions, the timing of medical interventions, and suggestions for adjusting such timing should be given and received in the proper cooperative spirit.

Finding the best balance between the correct treatment and allowing for as much sleep and restoration as possible shouldn't be an issue for anyone to lose sleep over.

Chapter 2

Doctors: The Good, The Bad, and the Totally Incomprehensible

Over the next two weeks Andrew continued to slowly improve in terms of his respiratory difficulties, gradually progressing from the intensive care unit to a regular pediatric medical ward. He did remain extremely weak, and made very little progress in his ability to move. Flush with renewed optimism after yet another recovery from terrible odds, Ruth and I easily attributed Andrew's lack of motor improvement to the simple prolonged effects of his recent battle against the RSV pneumonia. After all, even healthy adults and children are weakened after severe illness. His oxygen levels were getting better and better, and he no longer needed the inhaled respiratory therapy treatments (allowing a little more uninterrupted sleep at night).

We were also caught up in, but ultimately betrayed by, an unflagging sense of confidence that it was all temporary and fixable. Many parents may be overconfident about their baby's or child's illness out of the simple belief that "such things don't happen to us." It's an attitude perhaps similar to the detached interest with which Midwesterners view hurricanes on the East Coast or earthquakes in California. Terrible tragedies, hope they do okay, but won't change what I do because it's never going to happen here…

The fact is, most parents never really have the opportunity to see the storms that nature can unleash on the individual human body and so never contemplate the possibility of personal experience with severe illness until it happens. Newborn babies represent a wonderful, flawless beginning; most parents don't know of anyone whose children are in an intensive care unit (ICU) instead of in a home nursery.

Ruth and I, however, had seen it all—or at least thought we had. Because we were doctors, we knew what could happen, and we thus lived somewhat fearfully because of it. We were tripped up by the overconfidence of knowing too much. We knew Andrew's weakness was just a matter of recuperation because the facts, as *we* saw them, just didn't support anything else. His doctors weren't expressing the same optimism, but they obviously just didn't have the kind of insight we did. Looking back, I realize that even if parents know too little or too much, they aren't anywhere near prepared for what might happen to a child.

We contained our confidence, however, and agreed with Andrew's pediatrician and neurologist that a second opinion was still needed while Andrew remained in the hospital. The case was still not clear to the neurologist, and the implications of being wrong about weakness in a newborn were serious. Residents of Rhode Island, we were fortunately close to a mecca of medicine, Boston. On Andrew's neurologist's recommendation, we prepared to visit a hospital in Boston—Massachusetts General Hospital. As Harvard's premier institution, many in the medical profession joked that the initials really stood for Man's Greatest Hospital.

We gathered all the necessary information for the trip: pathology slides, X-ray films, discharge summaries, all the words and pictures that represented our baby's life. It all stood in stark contrast to the more mundane baby pictures, videos, and birth announcements that chronicle the beginning of life for most other newborns.

The day of Andrew's doctor appointment in Boston finally arrived. We dutifully checked over all the slides and X-ray films for the thousandth time, then kissed Andrew good-bye before he was to be transported hospital to hospital by ambulance. We followed in a car. The recent events must have shaken our indomitable faith in Andrew's positive outcome, because we both became increasingly nervous as we neared our destination.

Neither of us could eat much lunch, and instead we chose to hover outside the neurologist's office.

Andrew arrived shortly after we did, looking ridiculously small in the car seat that was strapped down to an adult-sized stretcher. The ambulance attendants had wrapped his head in a towel to keep him warm, which is also done to infirm, elderly patients who are brought to the hospital. The sight of a tiny baby dressed like a refugee from a nursing home would have been comical in other circumstances. And if we had known at that moment what we were destined to find out, that same resemblance to a nursing home resident would have been eerily prophetic, even sickening.

The neurologist finally waved us in. He was cordially aloof and asked questions about the pregnancy and birth, as well as Andrew's subsequent hospital courses in the Neonatal Intensive Care Unit and Pediatric Intensive Care Unit, in a professional, clinically detached manner. We were pinning our hopes on his expertise, however, and at the moment, warmth ranked far lower than knowledge on the priority scale. After speaking with us, he and Ruth went into another room to examine Andrew. I waited outside and listened to bells ringing and paper rustling. I heard Andrew cooing and occasionally crying. It seemed to be taking a very long time, and I didn't know if that was good or bad. Finally, I heard him tell Ruth to get him dressed.

The doctor then emerged and said very matter-of-factly, "I'd like to have a few of my residents come up and examine Andrew with me. I'll then need a few hours to go over the slides and X-rays. Why don't you both go down and get something to eat and come back around four o'clock?" When such words are spoken to parents who are also physicians—schooled in the ways of academic medicine—they became terrifying. In a teaching environment, doctors-in-training are best taught on actual patients who demonstrate rare or instructive physical findings. These particular characteristics may be classic for a certain disease. The characteristics may be sounds heard through a stethoscope, enlarged organs or nodes that are able to be felt, or visual abnormalities apparent to the eye or scope. For the physician or student lucky enough to observe it, an instructive physical exam is invaluable to a medical education. For the patient, however, demonstrating an instructive physical finding usually carries the same implications as being labeled a Great Case; it's bad. The majority of patients never realize the significance of all those residents standing in line to hear their heart murmur, or to elicit a reflex, or to feel their enlarged spleen. In fact, many patients feel good that they are able to help out young doctors, ignorant that such an opportunity is achieved by exposing diseased organs or short-circuited nerves to the detached groping of medical trainees.

Ruth and I definitely were not ignorant of these implications. As doctors, we had examined and appreciated our share of Great Cases. Yet this neurologist, whose job it was to determine if our child had a fatal neurologic disease and who knew we were doctors, could do nothing more than inform us he wished our son to teach his residents about some illuminating aspect of pediatric neurology. Dozens of questions raced through my mind. Did he want his residents to view Andrew because Andrew exhibited the classic symptoms of spinal muscular atrophy, or SMA, a fatal degenerative disease that had already been considered as one possible disease to explain my son's condition? Did Andrew simply have interesting findings that had no bearing on the neurologist's particular diagnosis? Did residents simply get called up routinely for any patient this doctor saw? Or did he want to demonstrate to his students how Andrew's other doctors had mistaken some findings that in actuality implied a more ominous disease? The more I thought about it, the more I felt that residents at such a high-powered institution wouldn't waste their time on something unless it were truly rare or educational—such as what physical findings belonging to a disease that struck infants, such as SMA, might represent.

I couldn't stand the crush of questions swirling around in my mind any longer. I struggled to sound as nonchalant as possible, but the question stuck in my throat at first. "So does Andrew have some interesting physical finding?" Not that I was particularly interested in any part of my son's physical examination, but I hoped I could get at least some clue as to why he had summoned his residents.

"I just want the residents to examine him with me. Why don't you both come back after I look at the slides?" he calmly responded, divulging nothing. *Do I have to beg, doctor?* I wanted to shout. It was maddening, but he had made it quite clear that further questioning would serve no useful purpose.

I felt sick to my stomach. Any confidence I had held in Andrew's health had vanished. A major breach had been opened in the fortress of conviction I had hidden behind, and suddenly nothing seemed certain anymore. Ruth and I picked up our coats and stumbled out of the office. As we exited the building, we looked at each other and knew we were thinking the same thing. We felt that he had told us very bad news, but until confirmation arrived in the form of Andrew's medical results, he preferred us to twist in the wind of uncertainty before telling us for sure.

We found refuge in our car, where we sat in the front seat and cried. The neurologist had done what any academic physician would have done when confronted by a patient with an interesting disease: he had done what we had been taught to do through years of medical school and residency. Yet as two parents, we felt that what we were being subjected to was nothing less than callous cruelty. We realized now how it was when one's entire future rested on the words of another, and those words were kept just out of reach. And so for the next hour or so we sat in the car. The minutes passed with frustrating slowness. We knew enough to agonize over the neurologist's every little word and action, but we still tried to cling to the hope left to us by not having been told horrible news for sure.

The time finally came: we had to return to the hospital. We wiped away our tears and trudged back. And we waited some more. My stomach began churning again. When the doctor finally came out and beckoned for us to follow him, by heart rate picked up. I could actually feel my face flush. We sat down in his office, Andrew having already begun the trip back to the hospital in Rhode Island by ambulance. We hadn't had a chance to tell him good-bye.

The neurologist looked at us across his desk and asked, "So what is your understanding of what has gone on?"

Calmly, as if I were discussing a patient's case on rounds, I answered, "Andrew's case is confusing. All the tests point to both a possible neuropathic process and a myopathic process. Either or both could be the primary disease, such as spinal muscular atrophy, or they could be due to intrauterine or birth asphyxia." Not bad for someone teetering on the brink of total emotional disintegration. I had just told him in his own terms that Andrew's nerves and muscles had abnormalities on all the tests, which could be due to one of those dreaded neurologic diseases, or could be due to injury and low oxygen during birth.

Even years later I can't explain why I responded to this doctor with such dispassionate, coldly clinical detachment. By that time I had already harbored deep resentment against such a demeanor. Perhaps the neurologist's manner up to that time had convinced me I would be given his time and consideration only if I proved myself a professional equal. Equal footing at that time, in medicine's academic center, meant a rational scientific discussion about my son, free of emotional baggage and distracting parental concerns.

Or maybe it was entirely my doing, an unconscious attempt to distance myself from the personal agony that all these tests, and diagnoses, and prognoses brought on. Where other parents might have retreated behind simple denial or anger, I possibly found it easier to hide behind sophisticated explanations and detached scientific reasoning. I obviously didn't even consider these questions at the time, and I can't answer them now. I accept, however, that it would have been better had I been less of doctor and more of a parent and spouse.

"That's a pretty good summary," he replied.

I exhaled in relief. Maybe he, too, could add nothing to the case. So far, so good. Emboldened, I asked, "So it's still hard to say if all this is the result of asphyxia [low oxygen] and could get better, or if it's some degenerative disease?" The million-dollar question, but stated casually, it was just another part of this collegial conversation we fellow doctors were having.

"No, I don't believe this can be attributed to asphyxia. He may have suffered that to a small degree, but I don't see how that can account for all the changes I see in the muscle," he responded firmly.

I was taken by surprise. That had been what our hopes had rested on. In two seconds, without batting an eyelash, he had said it wasn't so. If Andrew's problems weren't due to reversible asphyxia, then Andrew's condition must be due to a primary nerve problem such as SMA, fatal at this age, or to a primary muscular dystrophy, like Jerry's kids, and they also die. And that would mean....I could tell the words had hit Ruth too. It suddenly was very hot in the room, and my chest suddenly became so tight I couldn't inhale against the pressure.

"You don't think any of this can be attributed to asphyxia?" Ruth repeated my question, as if by asking over and over we would get him to realize that he had misspoken the first several times.

"No, the muscle looks too unorganized and diseased, and the clinical picture is not consistent with asphyxia at all," he again responded calmly.

Hope truly dies slowly—or desperation will always trump acceptance of a terrible truth. Whatever the motivations, Ruth asked, to my own ears sounding like she was pleading, "What about the elevated muscle enzymes and the elevated liver function tests? They supported some acute injury."

"Well, I'm not sure how to explain those abnormalities, but I don't think at all that this can be explained by birth asphyxia."

We were stunned. We were actually beyond stunned. Shocked, despairing, disbelieving—all these words only approach the description of our reaction. I couldn't even swallow. Ruth asked about Andrew's prognosis.

Deliberately, matter-of-factly, the neurologist answered, "It's hard to say for sure, but I don't think it is very good. The muscle on the pathology slide looked destroyed. Certainly if it is denervation disease, the prognosis is equally bad." By *denervation disease,* the doctor meant one of the diseases where nerves degenerate, such as SMA, which is one such illness in children. Amyotrophic lateral sclerosis, also known as ALS or Lou Gehrig disease, are the adult equivalents.

"What about life expectancy?" I asked without really wanting him to answer. Everything seemed unreal; I felt as if I were acting out a part in a play. I was asking a question that had become a cliché in so many medical dramas.

He steepled his fingers in front of him. "Most infants die within two years, but the course is variable, especially since the diagnosis here is not exactly clear. Some children can live many years, although that would be rare."

"Will he live long enough to have children?" I could hear my voice tremble.

"No."

"But you can't really tell us how long he *will* live?" I asked again. Without waiting for the answer I already knew, I added, "Given his life expectancy, what do you think we should do? What do most parents do?"

The neurologist looked animated for the first time in the conversation. He responded, "I think everything should be done for these children, as they may live for some time—"

"Feeding tube? Tracheostomy?" I interrupted, as only a parent who has artificially prolonged life for others could ask.

"Yes, I think everything should of course be done. As I said, the course is variable. Although most children die in one or two years, sometimes we are pleasantly surprised. In fact, we are following one child who has lived over two years, and she can even sit up. So there is every reason for hope."

Sit up? *Sit up?* I asked fearfully, "And if they live longer, do they gain strength or continue to get weaker?"

"Well, yes, they tend to weaken, especially as growth means more mass to try to move. But with aggressive care they can live for years, and some even gain certain milestones, as I've said." His tone and demeanor seemed oddly placid. If I hadn't been hearing the actual words, I would have thought he was discussing the natural history of an ankle fracture and whether to leave it alone or cast it. "Again, we do everything for these children, because their lives can be prolonged."

"What tends to become of the children who are kept alive?"

"It's not uncommon for contractures to occur and progress. This typically affects the spine as well, leading to scoliosis. Sometimes this can be severe, but putting the child in a brace can help."

The final straw. By *contractures,* he meant gradual deformity, if he didn't die first.

The news we had just been told was so bad, so unthinkable, that I think all we could do was to keep questioning him. Perhaps he would finally surrender and admit he had been wrong about the whole thing, that he was so sorry he had put us through all this for nothing. It wasn't conscious thought; it was the only defense we had. "So even if it's not spinal muscular atrophy, the prognosis is very bad?"

The neurologist darted a glance at his watch before answering flatly, "Yes, on the basis of all the evidence, there is a very poor prognosis."

"And probably fatal?"

"Yes."

The neurologist began gathering up the papers on his desk and made reference to sending everything along to Andrew's own neurologist and pediatrician in Rhode Island. The meeting was clearly over, at least for him. He made sure to tell us we were welcome to call him with any other questions or concerns that might come, all in the same calm, detached voice.

In the heat of the moment, we hated him. The stakes for us in this evaluation were overwhelming, but this neurologic court of last appeal had devoted more time to teaching residents than dealing with us. Years later, able to look back with calmer reflection, I'm not sure if that physician really deserved our venom. He had done what we came to him for: he had given us his honest assessment of Andrew's case and evaluated all the data. He had given us more of a definite prognosis than any of the doctors in

Rhode Island had been able to do. And after all, it wasn't his place to sit down and cry with us. He had presented his honest and learned opinion in a clinically detached manner.

Were we simply shooting the messenger, something that many patients and families can't help but doing? There are no villains or tangible causes to attack when people are confronted with a terminal illness. Irrational though it may be, physicians invested with the task of fixing that illness can become the most apparent scapegoats to bear the brunt of the understandable anger such a situation generates. Had we simply chosen an undeserving, innocent physician as the target of our fury and disbelief?

Ruth and I went on to receive equally horrendous news from other physicians, but we felt only gratitude at their compassion under such circumstances. I have been the unfortunate bearer of terrible news for many of my patients, and only rarely have I been met with anger directed at me or at my demeanor. Ruth and I may simply have been very difficult parents to confront in any way about anything. I feel that any parent will be less than rational when faced with very bad news about a child and should be given every possible benefit of every doubt. The neurologist was justified in keeping his message dignified and in keeping his comportment professionally detached. We resented, however, that he treated Andrew and us as extensions of the medical learning process and that he exhibited little empathy or compassion while giving a professional opinion. He only fulfilled a part of what physicians should offer patients. The easiest role of a physician is offering learned advice and facts about a medical condition. The hard part is doing so while keeping the patient's perspective in mind and remaining sensitive to the turmoil that confronting illness may promote.

Ruth and I literally stumbled out of the office and somehow wound up back in the car. Ruth took the wheel and we headed home to Rhode Island. While the chaos of Boston's rush hour swirled around us, we sat in silence and separately contemplated what we had heard. All I could think about was years of slow, painful disability, leading to deformity and possibly paralysis. That's if Andrew didn't succumb to the other possibility mentioned and died much sooner.

Visions of family outings flashed through my mind. Two kids out in front, followed by Mom and Dad wheeling an immobile, twisted Andrew along in his wheelchair, drawing stares from all the running and jumping kids surrounding us in the park. Or family outings *without* Andrew, pleasant on the surface but made possible by leaving a third child at home. And that third child wondering why he had been left at home—or worse, *knowing* why he had been left at home. Obviously, these images were melodramatic and irrational, but such musings became my reality in the growing darkness of the car during the ride home.

When these thoughts became too much to bear, I did the only thing that any parent-physician would do in such circumstances. I didn't put my arm around Ruth to comfort her. I didn't call our parents and explain what we now knew. I didn't try to calm us both down. No, I went straight to a medical textbook of neurologic disease that we had brought along. While Ruth drove, I sought to take over where all the other doctors had obviously failed or misdiagnosed. For the rest of the trip I sat paging through the book, jumping from chapters entitled "Muscle Dystrophies" to "Degenerative Nerve Diseases" to "Pediatric Disorders." Every so often, I would spot something that described something similar to Andrew's circumstances, something that had a much better prognosis. After reading the entire description of that particular disease, I'd invariably get excited that I'd hit upon the exact answer everyone else had overlooked. I think I learned more about muscular dystrophy during that car ride than during my entire four years of medical school.

So there we were on the lonely highway between Boston and Rhode Island, my wife straining to drive and watching the road through the tears, her husband thumbing frantically through a book of neurologic nightmares, occasionally lecturing her about the latest disorder than resembled Andrew's, as long as it had a better prognosis.

Now, of course, parent-physicians no longer have a monopoly on ready access to medical information. I wonder how many patients or parents of patients now rush home to the Internet and surf through various Websites in the same frenzied desperation with which I pawed through that textbook. I had ironically fallen into the same trap as the neurologist had: we had both forsaken the importance of comforting others while relying on cold, hard facts as the only solution to a family's anguish. Today's parents need not fall into the same trap. Seeking to confront tragic circumstances with knowledge is certainly admirable and may at times be of help. Offering crucial compassion and strength to loved ones, however, is definitely underrated next to the sometimes more unreliable support of the Internet, textbooks, or even physicians.

By the time we reached home, I had grown tired of chasing after textbook answers, and we were both tired of just about everything. I made it to the bedroom before sinking to the floor, sobbing. I remember pleading with Andrew's pediatrician on the phone that night to please help us, that she had to somehow help us. If there was a bottom to our lives up to that point, through Andrew's difficulties right after his birth and even the roller coaster rides through the ICUs, I had hit it.

Despite the neurologist's assessment, we remained unsatisfied after the debacle in Boston and had asked Andrew's pediatrician to find yet another pediatric neurologist who could provide a reliable third opinion. The closest one we could find was located in New York City. That was terrifying enough to someone born and raised in the Midwest. But we had not taken Andrew on a trip of any length since he was born, and all we could imagine was some catastrophe happening on the road. Boston had been less than an hour away. Would his airway collapse because of poor positioning in his car seat? Would he suddenly choke and aspirate in the back seat, leaving us on the highway with a dead baby? When the worst had already happened, nothing seemed too ridiculous or improbable to us.

We resigned ourselves to the trip no matter how many nightmares were imagined, but this time it was not because we were desperately seeking a new opinion to contradict the prognosis we had been given. We were only hoping that this new specialist could at least give us a diagnosis, instead of leaving us in a limbo of "something very bad" or "maybe a slow and lingering death; but maybe not." Even if he confirmed SMA, thus pronouncing a virtual death sentence, at least we would know. So again we dutifully placed Andrew in his car seat, brought all the records and X-ray films, and set off for our next encounter with the Medical Establishment. Our own profession had gone from trusted institution to fearsome stranger.

The trip to New York was uneventful. We wound up in the Bronx at the Albert Einstein School of Medicine. We walked in the door of the latest specialist's office, and we were met with the sight of a young couple pushing a baby in a baby carriage ahead of them. Both had red, swollen eyes, and the baby's mother was still crying. Ruth and I looked at other. That same sick feeling started churning in my stomach.

We were again shown to an examining room, where we readied ourselves for the next assault on our lives. It was unbelievable that only two months could reverse a decade of collegial acceptance and fellowship and generate such resentment on our part. It's natural and understandable for parents to seek out someone to blame for a situation that has occurred without cause or reason, and what better scapegoats than the very people who kept giving us the worst news we had ever received? Nonetheless, I maintain that Andrew's illness only lowered our threshold of tolerance for insensitivity; it did not unjustly create insensitivity out of an otherwise humane and compassionate experience.

Our mood was therefore grim, unforgiving, and defensive as we waited for Dr. S, the latest neurologist. Then the door opened, and a pudgy, pleasant, gray-haired grandfather walked in and apologized for being late. This unpretentious little man introduced himself as Dr. S. This was the learned pediatric physician, the absolute pinnacle of neuromuscular disease specialists? He looked and sounded as if he'd be more at home behind a delicatessen counter preparing a pastrami on rye. My doubts grew as he smiled widely and asked if he could see our "little fella."

However, he quickly asserted his expertise as he asked us probing questions about Andrew's birth and his subsequent course of illness. He then asked us to undress Andrew so he could examine him. I was instantly horrified at the thought of being in the room while my son was again subjected to a neurologist's examination, being forced to watch as all of Andrew's disabilities were starkly put on display. I turned from the exam table and pretended to look for something in Andrew's baby bag—anything so I wouldn't have to watch.

Dr. S, though, couldn't have been kinder or more caring than if he actually had been Andrew's grandfather. Each maneuver or reflex hammer tap was accompanied by soothing words and a gentle touch. Andrew was taken from Ruth's arms only once: Dr. S held Andrew up in front of a window and stared at his face intently for several minutes. Afterward, he told us to get Andrew dressed. And that was that. We all came out of it relieved, with dignity intact.

Now came the moment of truth. Dr. S sat us down and came right to the point. He told us he was "95% sure" Andrew had SMA, type 1.

Bang. That was it.

A brief, almost electric jolt went through my body at his words, but I felt no overwhelming panic, no urge to scream out in disbelief, no rage. Admittedly, we had already been given a very good idea of what the meeting could result in by the neurologist in Boston; he had knocked the initial hole in our wall of denial. But my calm acceptance of Andrew's fatal diagnosis had to be because of more than that. It's true that if you tear a Band-Aid off quickly, all at once, the pain is never quite as bad or lingering than if you were to nudge it off bit by bit. Many times my patients barely feel the sting of a needle if I inject them quickly and without build-up, instead of trying the puncture slowly and carefully.

Maybe the same goes for receiving terrible news about a loved one. Undoubtedly, however, the pain may have been deadened just a little by Dr. S's calm, compassionate approach. He addressed us directly, always looking right at us, appearing as though he were personally invested in how we were receiving his words, instead of simply trying to choose his words carefully and cautiously.

And finally, perhaps deep down, I was spared crippling anguish or panic by an actual involuntary sense of relief instead. SMA is divided into three types on the basis of the age at onset. Andrew apparently had type 1, which presents before six months of age and is invariably fatal by age two or three years. I imagine that the slow, lingering, crippling, deforming, painful life the Boston neurologist had described, all leading to eventual death anyway, terrified me more than the thought of an early death, one we hoped could be made comfortable. Perhaps at times like this, there is no stereotypical behavior for a parent, no rational explanation for why a situation is perceived in a certain way. This was my first realization of medicine's lack of absolutes.

In any case, Dr. S went on to gently elaborate on why he felt the way he did. He told us he had seen "tongue fasciculations" on Andrew. *Fasciculation* is a term describing a continuous twitching or squirming of a particular muscle. Internal medicine physicians such as myself usually had read about it, but only very occasionally are such findings seen. It usually occurred in the large muscles of the leg in certain diseases and would always warrant summoning in the residents and students to hungrily view a Great Physical Finding.

I had never seen fasciculations of a patient's tongue, nor had I ever even thought to look. It is apparently pathognomonic (that is, virtually diagnostic of) SMA, and it is most easily seen under direct sunlight. That explained why Dr. S had held Andrew up in front of the window for so long. It astonished me to hear that one simple, observed physical finding had perhaps told more than the thousands of dollars' worth of tests we had been through. Other aspects of Andrew's muscular weakness supported the diagnosis of SMA as well, according to Dr. S. There were certain confusing aspects that didn't fit in with SMA, such as the presence of reflexes in his legs, and certain parts of the muscle biopsy were confusing as well.

All in all, though, Dr. S was reasonably certain Andrew did indeed have SMA, also known as the disease from hell.

As if to underscore his belief in the diagnosis, Dr. S went on to ask us if we had banked some of Andrew's blood at a special genetic testing lab. You see, he explained, infants with SMA can die very suddenly at any time. It would be important to have some of Andrew's blood available, because in the future, a definite genetic test for SMA could be perfected. In other words, confirming the diagnosis even after Andrew had died would help our peace of mind and could have implications for any future children or grandchildren. Tears started welling up hotly in my eyes as I heard these words. Talking about my own child in the past tense drove home the reality of the situation more than anything else had up to then.

But the hard part hadn't even been touched on yet. Dr. S delicately explained that parents react differently when faced with the future of a child like Andrew. He told us that some chose to never give in, despite the bleak future. They were parents who loved and comforted their children and fought for their children's lives with tracheostomies, ventilators, feeding tubes—whatever it took. Other parents accepted the inevitability of the disease. These parents provided comfort and love, but they had different ideas about quality of life versus quantity of life, and these parents chose not intervene as nature took its course.

Strangely, I began feeling a sense of relief rather than horror, even though we were discussing Andrew's life and death. Sadness and despair gripped me, to be sure. The lump in my throat and the tears I couldn't blink back betrayed the presence of those emotions. Yet we were being told by this authority that assuring Andrew's comfort and happiness, if even for a short time, could be as noble a goal as any caring parent could want for their child.

Ruth and I had taken care of many people who lived their lives tethered to tubes and catheters. Whether it was those experiences or our independent belief that existing through machines and artificial means is not what life is intended to be for a child, we knew it was not what we wanted for

Andrew. Dr. S was telling us that such a decision was okay, considering the diagnosis—not right and not wrong, because this issue was a very personal one and one based on intangibles that differed from family to family. For us, it we felt it was the best decision we could make for our son, given the genes he had been dealt.

We talked of not starting tube feedings should Andrew become unable to eat on his own. Again, Dr. S told us that if done mercifully, always with Andrew's comfort in mind, this could also be seen as letting nature take its inevitable course. It was a discussion I'd had with patients' families before, less commonly with the patients themselves. I felt now an odd sense of disconnection as I discussed planning for my own son's death. There was no hysteria or angry outbursts from Ruth or me, only unhurried, accepting words and questions.

Perhaps we had been given enough time to come to terms with the truth since Boston. We had come to New York no longer in total denial, and so we were probably able to cope better. But we were confronting for the first time an unequivocal opinion of our son's fatal diagnosis. I feel strongly that the humane, patient, and empathetic manner in which Dr. S presented this awful truth, and his willingness to accept our feelings and decisions while giving us his own honest feelings, did much to keep Ruth and me from totally disintegrating, as we had before, in Boston. He used but did not hide behind cold medical facts and terms. He didn't leave us to simply choose between life-altering decision A or B with no guidance. Nor did he promote his own opinions regarding the sanctity of life at whatever cost as the only acceptable option.

That day we chose not to prolong the inevitable death of our child. With Dr. S's kind support and his assurance of the diagnosis of SMA, Ruth and I actually felt more at peace than we had felt since Andrew's birth. We still felt incredibly sad, terribly empty—but we felt at peace. And if we promised to make his death as comfortable and painless as possible, we owed it to Andrew and to ourselves to make his life as satisfying and as happy as possible as well.

After recommending one last specialized X-ray film to lay any lingering diagnostic doubts to rest, Dr. S wished us all the best and told us we could call him any time, at his office or at his home. I didn't know then if such concern was offered because we three were all part of the medical fraternity or because of his genuine sympathy for those in our position. I'm sure now that Dr. S is simply a very good and kind person and feels such empathy toward all his patients and their parents.

Ruth and I drove away secure in the realization that our baby had a terminal disease; and we understood the tears of the parents pushing their baby in a stroller we had seen on the way in. Nonetheless, we felt as if a huge weight had been lifted from us. Never would I have believed that a terminal neurologic disease in one of our children could become reality; nor would I have believed that such a reality would have inspired anything other than anguish and hopelessness. But now I was living that unimaginable reality, and I was accepting it with peaceful resignation.

Being left with the unknown may allow just enough room for hope to still linger; finally knowing the truth, despite the pain, allows acceptance to begin, and one can start moving on—not that any of us actually have a choice. But for our family, finally knowing the truth may indeed have dashed any hope for any actual recovery. It did, however, grant us hope for healing.

Us Versus Them

Doctors and lawyers: you can't live with 'em, you can't live without 'em. Almost by definition, someone must be going through medical, financial, or legal misfortune to warrant the help of a doctor or lawyer. Essentially, doctors benefit from the loss or impairment of that most precious gift: one's health. Doctors are also the professionals who can dispassionately put people through costly and often uncomfortable procedures. They can assert that those procedures won't be too uncomfortable while remaining well out of reach of those well-intentioned tortures themselves. Perhaps these are some of the reasons many people view doctors as "them": "*they* ordered such-and-such a test"; "did *they* tell you any results yet?" "*they* said it was nothing to worry about"; "*they* make you wait so long."

As a physician, I had attempted to understand this point of view, but deep down, I had considered such opinions as inappropriately antagonistic and unappreciative. "They" weren't a group of unfeeling, socially inept conspirators, plotting ways of obtaining the greatest amount of money while spending as little time as possible doing so. "They" included me—healers who can't always live up to the unreasonable expectations of their patients.

Now, however, I found myself in a position exemplifying what some would regard as poetic justice: a formerly omnipotent physician suddenly reduced to just another desperate, dependent family member coping with a serious medical problem. Perhaps *The Doctor,* starring William Hurt, was so successful because it appealed to the public's desire to see such irony visited upon a physician. *The Doctor* tells the story of an unfeeling, egotistical doctor who remained an unsympathetic character up until he was diagnosed with the same form of cancer he had diagnosed in his own patients. Only when faced with the prospect of dying and having to endure a tracheostomy did he see the light and became compassionate, and he was a better person for it.

Our experience with Andrew taught us that the message of that movie—how a callous physician turned patient and thus was transformed into kind and caring person and doctor—was far too simplistic and self-righteous. Unfortunately, we found such a portrayal not completely unrealistic, either. Throughout Andrew's life, our most agonizing and our most comforting moments have both come at the hands of our fellow physicians.

Part of my own discomfort with the medical profession resulted from my own particular experience. I was condemned to endure the irony that as a pulmonologist, or lung specialist, I would have to watch my own son die a pulmonary death. It was a process I was all too familiar with, one I was well schooled in the ways of preventing. An even greater irony was that several of my colleagues took care of patients in whom rapid death had been prevented by artificial and prolonged ventilation. Going to work and talking with my colleagues, then, denied me any possible escape from the future facing us—and in fact drove it home in vivid detail.

The most painful example of this occurred shortly after I had started back to work following our trip to New York. One of my more cerebral colleagues came into my office and asked what was going on with Andrew. I reluctantly mentioned the diagnosis of SMA (the words never stopped sticking my throat).

"Do you know if it's type 1, 2, or 3?" he asked.

I was surprised. I had never known there were three types before Dr. S had informed us during our visit with him, but here, one of my partners was better informed.

"It's, um, probably type 1, but we still don't know absolutely for sure," I muttered feebly, uncomfortable talking about the specifics of my son's terminal illness.

He continued on in his usual authoritative, matter-of-fact tone. "You know, I'm following a kid with SMA. He's actually getting ready to graduate from high school."

My heart rate must have tripled; I could feel my face growing hot. *Graduate high school? With SMA?* Almost nonchalantly, he went on, "Yeah, must weigh about 90 pounds, and he's sort of twisted up because of his contractures, but he still gets around pretty well in his wheelchair—"

"He's got a trach in though, right?" I interrupted anxiously.

"No, believe it or not, he's never required a permanent trach. He has been intubated once or twice though. His lung capacity is incredibly small, but since he doesn't move around much and had almost no body mass, he's never required long-term ventilation."

I was feeling lightheaded and short of breath, but I managed to mumble an embarrassingly lame excuse to end the conversation. He appeared oblivious to the turmoil I had been thrown into and wished me and my family good luck before leaving unconcernedly. I immediately slumped in my chair and dissolved into total panic and despair. Part of me tried dwelling on the facts that this patient had both survived to graduate from high school and remained productive.

Soon, however, the thought that swirled around and around in my mind, that bit and gnawed at me, was only that he had survived. This was the future for my child? Did he really think his description would make me feel better? Would he care to imagine such a future for his two beautiful little daughters? That kid had been afflicted with the same thing that Andrew had, yet had lived indefinitely without ever needing a tracheostomy, slowly becoming more and more a prisoner of his own body. We had finally reconciled ourselves to, and had prepared ourselves for, the fact that Andrew was supposed to die, not linger and eventually become a human pretzel.

A sudden realization stopped my silent ranting like a slap in the face. I was actually becoming panic-stricken at the thought that my son might not die prematurely after all. I was enraged that someone would try to encourage me with stories of people such as my son graduating from high school because I might have to deal with protracted disability and struggle instead of a painful but mercifully short time to death. What the hell had happened to me? What the hell kind of a parent, or person, was I really? My head was throbbing and my chest was tightening, as if I were drowning on dry land.

I closed the door and consciously took several deep breaths, but I felt no more calm. When I could stand the anxiety no longer, I first called my well-meaning colleague and asked him for the name of his patient so I could review the patient's medical records. I then called Dr. S in New York and left a message for him to page me as soon as possible.

That catastrophe fortunately resolved without too much more agonizing. The patient I had been told of had been diagnosed with SMA type 2, which apparently has a later age at onset and can indeed lead to chronic disability instead of premature death. Dr. S also called me back and assured me that he foresaw no such future for Andrew, since there was no doubt my son was affected by type 1. Of course, unspoken but in his voice nonetheless was a hint of uncertainty, an implicit provision: "assuming Andrew really does have SMA, he would have type 1." At the time, I couldn't dwell on what he wasn't saying. I was too busy feeling relieved at what he actually did tell me. I had prepared myself for the premature death that would happen after all.

Next to the experience in Boston, that episode stands out as the worst encounter with my own profession. It was not the only one, however. Another of my colleagues made sure to point out to me that he also was taking care of a patient with SMA, one who had also survived into adulthood. I cut the conversation short before he could even start to describe his patient's appearance and lifestyle. These weren't cruel people. They actually had very good professional reputations as both clinicians and as compassionate healers. So why were their attempts at empathy so insensitive and hurtful? As a doctor, was I expected to divest myself of all my personal baggage and view my personal situation with detached clinical perspective?

The answers weren't there. I certainly had no previous experience to guide me, nor did I know of any physicians who had been similarly afflicted. I did know that I had become a parent first and a doctor a distant second. I started dreading meetings with any fellow physicians who might have their own stories to tell of professional encounters with neurologic disease. Andrew was not the next Grand Rounds case to speculate about; he was my son.

Even Andrew's own pediatrician exhibited discomforting changes in support and communication. On the one hand, she went above and beyond the call of duty. In my experience, few general pediatricians would so willing take on such an enormous amount of responsibility. She personally supervised a child who had not only baffled many of the best neurologic specialists available but who was also felt to be terminally ill and who was predicted to only deteriorate. She arranged repeated second opinions and stood by us through tough and controversial personal decisions. All in a day's work for any conscientious pediatrician? Perhaps it should be, but we have only rarely enjoyed such unswerving responsibility since.

At other times, communication with Andrew's pediatrician resulted in unintended pain. While discussing the pros and cons of Andrew receiving a painful polio vaccine, she mused nonchalantly that nobody would even know if he actually ever came down with polio anyway, given his already profound weakness. After almost every examination, she would ask if we also thought Andrew's head seemed to be getting molded from lying in one position for so long. Each time she thought out loud, which Ruth interpreted as, "Don't you feel as though your son is becoming more deformed with each passing day?", required almost a week for Ruth to recover from.

On balance, our pediatrician's actions more than outweighed what unintentional pain her words may have caused. And in our frantic state of mind, we undoubtedly became mired in words we could have otherwise risen above or brushed off. We instead resented those words and allowed them to fester, almost as if we were looking for easy external scapegoats to absorb the anger and wretchedness we had no one else to blame for. I have ever since remained acutely aware of the power my words could have over patients already coping with illness or difficult circumstances.

Most of the time, though, we were alienated from members of our own profession by more casual encounters. During Andrew's hospital stay, numerous doctors who knew either Ruth or me would greet us in the hall or walk into Andrew's room unannounced, and without preamble would ask, "So, have they found a diagnosis yet?" Certainly a reasonable question to pose to a colleague about an unrelated patient. But it was our son that diagnosis mattered to, not a detached Excellent Teaching Case. And they were directly asking his parents.

Each clumsy intrusion made us feel as if we were the caretakers of nothing more than a specimen valuable to medical science instead of the parents of a newborn baby. Often, questions of pure medical curiosity and explanations of scientific fact and trivia were thrown out in reply to our predicament. Words of genuine caring were rarely heard.

In my experience, such a response to personal misfortune or tragedy is not uncommon among physicians. Such professional demeanor allows us to succeed well in medical school, where we score points for our incisive renditions of medical facts and observations. There is neither the time nor the interest on medical rounds for discussion about how a patient is coping, or how unfortunate a particular situation actually is. Such an intense focus on scientific fact serves physicians well through the rigors of residency and academic medical pursuits.

Perhaps confronting serious or tragic illness with clinical explanations of medical fact offers a physician convenient refuge. There are few words that can alleviate the pain and anxiety a patient or family member suffers. There are rarely answers to "why?" But there are always explanations of processes, theories on physiology, and educated guesses as to diagnoses that provide concrete answers—or at least plausible explanations. Responding to inexplicable tragedy with irrefutable medical information offers a physician the opportunity to say something—anything—and to provide some positive impact. We were given such so-called solace by friends and even relatives who were also doctors. There was never a shortage of speculation on details of Andrew's muscle biopsies. Simple understanding and empathy were in much shorter supply. The comfort provided by professional expertise and knowledge is magnified, and for most of us is much more valuable, when softened by compassionate words and attitude.

I do not mean to suggest that a physician can know when and how to offer such words of compassion only if he or she has experienced personal medical hardship. To advocate such a view, I would have to believe that people in general, be they teachers, physicians, or parents, can't be understanding and empathic individuals without experiencing situations they are responsible for. This obviously is an extreme requirement for successfully negotiating life's encounters and obligations. Moreover, prior experiences may be so intense that they only prevent objectivity and promote inappropriate resentment when similar circumstances are confronted later. I can certainly attest to this pitfall on a personal level.

Particular insights did arise, however, out of living both inside and outside the white coat. Such perspectives drove the desire to write this book. Compassion and empathy are by no means created by personal experience, but they may be sharpened by it. Doctors do not have to go home each night to a child with a disability in order to administer compassionate treatment of patients. When inspecting the plaques on a physician's office wall, I wouldn't recommend walking out if a hospital discharge summary isn't displayed among them. In negotiating the complicated course through childhood illness, however, special insights forged from direct experience may just add a little further delicacy to handling a situation.

Communication

The interactions between physicians and patients, or between physicians and parents of children who are patients, may largely determine how a family copes with profound tragedy. I have learned more about this relationship as the parent of a seriously ill infant than I have learned from over a decade of serving patients as their physician. The relationship between health care provider and patient or family cannot become strained by anger, misunderstanding, or suspicion. It is important for parents to realize and accept that such passionate reactions are not always justified. Health care providers, however, must also respect their responsibility to keep those emotions from igniting.

Looking back, I am almost ashamed, and certainly remorseful, at how unjustified some of my thoughts and reactions toward my son's physicians were at the beginning and continue to be now. The preceding narrative of my attempts to cope with news of Andrew's true condition is not embellished or exaggerated. My wife and I came to actually perceive as the enemy any physician who dared voice a pessimistic opinion about Andrew's eventual outcome. Conversely, the doctors who optimistically maintained that he was suffering from a totally reversible, benign disease immediately won our trust and admiration.

Both types of physicians were generally supportive and compassionate in their dealings with us; it was their actual message that provoked our antagonism or trust. Essentially, then, we began trusting only those physicians whose message we liked, and we felt alienated by bearers of more sobering news or opinions, even if they communicated an honest, informed message. To Ruth and me, the thought that our son could have a serious or terminal illness was so horrifying that any physician who believed in such a possibility deserved resentment and couldn't really be trusted.

As irrational as this behavior was, it becomes even more remarkable considering that Ruth and I are both physicians ourselves—putting us in a position that is neither a curse nor a blessing but rather one that should have granted us particular insight and perspective. Nonetheless, in the space of several very short, but at the same time very long, months, we went from trustful, secure insiders to mistrustful, antagonistic parents alienated from our physician colleagues. So how must it be for the majority of parents who probably have only limited experience with the medical establishment before their world caves in around them and their seriously ill child?

It is probably even easier for parents with little prior connection to medicine to take out their frustrations and anger on the bearer of bad news: the physician. As a doctor who has been on the receiving end of such behavior, and as a parent who has fallen into this trap, I can acknowledge that it is unfortunately understandable. Confronting the possibility of a child's suffering, or even death, is the most stressful situation a parent may face. Such stress almost inevitably leads to irrational blame and reactions, misunderstanding, and misinterpretation.

Can anything be done about this unfortunate set of circumstances? Yes. First, parents need to be reassured that feelings of resentment or distrust are an understandable reaction when the parents receive unexpected bad news about a child. When the unimaginable occurs, parents don't have the luxury of time to look back and realize that doctors would be irresponsible if they didn't deliver as knowledgeable and as honest an opinion as they are able. Second, physicians should accept such a reaction as only one manifestation of parental grief and not take it as a personal attack on their wisdom or integrity. Taking it personally, and responding in kind with indignation, makes a bad situation worse, and this does say something about that physician's integrity. It took my experiences as a parent for me to realize the value of a composed, compassionate response to uncontrollable emotion.

Bottom line: parents confronting a child's severe illness or death are entitled to a great deal of leeway in terms of coming to grips with bad news. All the conscientiousness in the world may still be overshadowed by grief and unreasonable antagonism. On the other hand, it remains the physician's prime responsibility to inform the truth regardless. The importance of how that truth is delivered cannot be overstated, as exemplified by Dr. S. He gave us perhaps the worst news a parent could hear. And yet we left him almost grateful. We had at least finally been told the definite truth. And for the first time, we didn't feel alone. We had someone who genuinely seemed to care, and he was a scientist as well. This was a doctor who realized that such news required more than a little compassion to deliver. This one meeting generated trust that could not be voided, even when he would eventually be proven wrong in both his diagnosis and prognosis for Andrew.

Conversely, bad news delivered in a less than compassionate manner can provoke very justified resentment and anger on a parent's part. Most of my encounters with the medical profession reinforced my pride at being a member of that profession. Too many of our experiences, however, instead confirmed the stereotype of the insensitive, cold clinician. Even more disillusioning, such negative interactions came when my wife and I were recognized as fellow physicians, able to converse with and understand at the same level as Andrew's caregivers. How must it be for parents and family members with no prior relationship to the medical establishment, with little or no sophistication when it comes to illness, technology, or science?

Doctors, or any health care professional, almost by definition have little control over the messages they must deliver. During one muscular dystrophy clinic appointment, a nurse practitioner talked to Andrew and me about his overall health. In the midst of advice about flu shots and tips for good nutrition, she nonchalantly asked, "And if next winter Andrew develops a very serious respiratory infection, would you want everything done for him? We do have machines that could breathe for him."

Essentially, I was being asked if I wanted all lifesaving measures taken or if I would prefer that my child be allowed to die peacefully were he to become very ill. My first paranoid thought was that something must have been discovered during that visit to make her feel the need to ask such a question, some lab test or physical finding that told them Andrew was going to die sooner than expected. It took frenzied phone calls and hours of agitated worry before I was convinced that it had only been brought up as a matter of routine for a child with Andrew's disease.

My anxiety then turned to anger as I remembered the nurse practitioner's casual tone. My son's possible death was thrown out like an afterthought, as if we had been discussing the pros and cons of toilet training. The motive behind the question had admittedly been appropriate, as was the need for knowing our wishes. The timing, the communication, though, were all wrong—and hurtful.

Many times since then, I have had to ask other family members that same question, sometimes even over the phone. Speaking of a loved one's death, or asking someone to take responsibility for determining that death, is unfortunately made necessary by the gravity of so many illnesses. It can't help but be painful no matter how it's handled. The pain and the memories of that experience linger long after but can at least be numbed by sensitivity to ensuring the proper time of and the proper preparation for confrontation. The implications of asking a parent whether a child should be kept alive or allowed to die mercifully can obviously be devastating. Even discussing a child's illness short of considerations of life or death can be emotionally exhausting. To bring these issues up into an otherwise routine discussion, or to broach them at a time of convenience for the physician, can be shocking, demeaning, and disheartening. It was for me.

Justifiable apprehension and anger over an insensitive approach certainly does not have to be limited to extreme life or death issues. Discussing test results, defining future limitations or disabilities, or simply predicting how long a child's hospitalization will last can all give rise to a huge amount of parental anxiety. Gentle communication can go a long way toward soothing the pain and frustration surrounding a sick child. Even seemingly innocuous news may be magnified by childhood illness.

Finally, communication cannot be complete without simple listening, an extremely underrated quality under even unexceptional conditions. Medical practice lends itself especially poorly to the act of listening to the other side, given the increasing numbers of patients, the incessant demands of office and hospital responsibilities, and the diminishing amount of time that can be allotted. Taking in a parent's frustrations without intervening results in few tangible or, to be blunt, reimbursable, outcomes. Unfortunately, then, listening has become regarded as an expendable obligation. It is anything but, especially when a child's circumstances become so tragic as to make any attempt at words meaningless.

Some reading this may be tempted to respond with, "Well, *du-u-uh*..." Indeed, for someone to acknowledge the importance of insightful words and sensitive listening in the course of providing instruction about professional medical care would appear on the surface to be unnecessary. Drawing upon my own experiences, and in speaking with other parents and patients alike, such considerations are not superfluous. For some health care professionals, these considerations are simply pushed too far down the ladder of priorities in favor of science and dispassion.

A physician should not be reluctant to recognize when an approach has been inappropriate. Setting pride aside and learning from unfortunate behavior will promote eventual healing, regardless of the actual medical outcome. This is not meant as a condescending indictment against doctors in general, most of whom still manage to demonstrate humane communication with patients despite long hours and unimaginable stress. It is instead intended as an acknowledgment of mistakes committed and lamentable discussions made with patients during my own experiences as a physician, brought into clearer perspective from my experiences as a parent.

The bearer of bad news is as much one's professional responsibility as is treating that bad news; taking care of *how* it is communicated is as much a part of that responsibility as is seeing to *what* is actually said.

Second Opinions

For most people, the only thing more valuable than their own health is the health of their children. Accordingly, when a child's health is threatened to the point of requiring intensive care, I feel that no reasonable effort should be spared to assure a good outcome. Most opinions and plans of action voiced by a physician during critical illness carry serious, often life-and-death implications. Under such extreme conditions, a second informed opinion may provide peace of mind and the acknowledgment that a recommended course of action is indeed the best under the circumstances. Furthermore, a second opinion may help reinforce reality to parents deep in denial, parents who might otherwise be tempted to avoid the inevitable and waste valuable time. This is not to say that second opinions should automatically always be requested. With respect to critically ill children, virtually any decision or clinical action may have tremendous repercussions. Second-guessing several decisions can delay crucial interventions and would certainly frustrate and alienate the very care providers who are trying to achieve a successful result. Moreover, second, third, or even fourth opinions will rarely erase the reality of unpleasant or disheartening illness.

All too often, however, diagnoses and prognoses are not straightforward. Andrew's entire life can attest to this. Difficult choices may need to be made on less than definite information. In these circumstances, a parent should never feel too intimidated or too unsure to ask for a second opinion. In the same light, a physician should never feel slighted or mistrusted. There is never cause for ego to take precedence over the need for parents and doctors alike to do whatever is necessary to achieve the best possible outcome and to assure as much peace of mind as possible.

As a physician, I had previously felt somewhat uncomfortable when one of my patients asked for another opinion. I regarded such a request as evidence of inadequacy on my part, or as evidence of a patient seeking only good news, not reality. I became the parent of a critically ill child, however, whose course was so confusing that specialists called in second opinions without waiting for our request. It became much easier to accept that even the best of doctors cannot know everything.

Of course, Ruth and I did ask for several additional consultations at various stages in my son's illness. Yet we still continued to trust in Andrew's original physician implicitly. The uncertainty surrounding Andrew's diagnosis meant my son's life, with little hope for a second chance in the future. I consider that to varying degrees, any serious health problem should be managed with the same attitude; one usually gets only one chance to ensure the future. Parents are burdened enough with the reality of coping with a child in the ICU, or with facing years of a child with a chronic disease. They don't deserve the extra burden of guilt or self-doubt over the advisability or etiquette of seeking more help.

Of course, there are downsides to second or third or however many alternative medical opinions are felt necessary. The risk of introducing a totally unexpected conclusion is quite real and may create even more disheartening uncertainty in parents' minds. More tests may be recommended, which may put the child through even more discomfort and which could uncover information that would only open up new avenues for confusion. Many laypeople feel that with its intensive medical school training, sophisticated technology, and ever-advancing medical research, current medical practice is always an exact science. Correct answers to difficult problems will therefore be arrived at if one's physician is smart enough or perseveres enough. Conversely, when a correct diagnosis isn't reached and a child can't be helped, a particular physician just hasn't pursued the problem in enough depth or hasn't had the benefit of proper training. Such beliefs make second opinions appealing and hopeful.

Sometimes second opinions actually fulfill expectations. I have seen instances in which a review of a confusing case by specialists actually resulted in a different diagnosis with entirely different implications. A fresh look by doctors not bogged down in weeks of frustration with the patient may result in a new theories or directions. In other cases, referral to an outside center is made because new or little-used treatments are not found elsewhere. Unfortunately, this happy set of circumstances tends to be the exception. The truth is, medicine really is much more of an art than an exact science. My son was subjected to all the sophisticated tests available, several different surgical attempts to secure a diagnosis, and several second opinions among doctors in three states, all of which was orchestrated by parents who, as doctors, thought they knew all the right questions to ask. Yet unbelievably, we remained without even a diagnosis, much less any treatment plan. It wasn't a situation born of medical malpractice or physician stupidity. It was indicative of the current state of medical practice that existed despite all the miraculous advances, medications, and discoveries trumpeted on the news. Answers aren't always possible, no matter who examines the patient. More frequently, second opinions open up differing physicians' philosophies on treating complicated issues as opposed to new medical facts or diagnoses.

As I stated previously, I had felt somewhat uncomfortable, if not resentful, when patients had requested a second opinion during the course of my treatment. I have come to realize, however, how intimidating human illness can be, and how fallible modern medical practice remains despite all the technological advances. I have dealt with many consultants in the years since Andrew's birth and have definitely appreciated the security of having supporting opinions in difficult cases. I have also dealt with many consultants as a parent and can express the same appreciation of the security their opinions brought with respect to Andrew's illness. I feel we did the right thing by leaving no stone unturned, no possibility overlooked.

I can also attest that as parents, we were at times turned inside out with frustration by the different diagnoses and different attitudes that were thrown at us by the very second opinions we had insisted on. Because medicine is an art as well as a science, health care professionals practice their specialties with certain differences. If parents accept that these expected differences can create pitfalls out of the most well-intentioned consultations, then they are well within their rights to call in second opinions in unusual or complicated cases. If those opinions result in nothing more than peace of mind, even that should be considered an admirable and worthy achievement when a child is critically ill.

Academic (Teaching) Hospitals: Should Sick Kids Ever Be the Lesson Plan?

Most pediatric ICUs, and certainly all neonatal ICUs, are located in large referral academic medical centers. Sooner or later, then, parents will run into the academic medical establishment. As a product of academic medical practice, I had been one of the strongest proponents of the value of passing on medical knowledge while practicing medicine. My son's illness completely changed that attitude.

I became resentful of what I perceived as other doctors putting teaching ahead of caring, of reducing the most heartbreaking tragedy in a parent's life to nothing more valuable than an excellent teaching opportunity. Using patients as educational examples came to appear almost demeaning. I became in fact so affected that I could no longer function as an academic physician; teaching medical students and residents on the backs of patients became virtually repulsive. It was the major force behind my decision to uproot my family and change to a private practice in which I was allowed to treat patients exclusively without teaching responsibilities. Now the turmoil has settled somewhat, allowing me to take more objective views of my experiences and of the role of academics in the treatment of patients in general and of sick children in particular.

Academic medical centers are by definition hospitals that are used by and staffed by medical schools; they are thus integral parts of medical training programs. These institutions tend to be major referral centers for patients requiring intensive or specialized care. Because they participate in medical education, these hospitals are staffed by trainees around the clock, usually in the form of medical students, interns, and residents. Critically ill patients therefore have access to close observation and intervention at any time without waiting for a physician to come in from home. For children who can deteriorate or change drastically within minutes (an all-too-common characteristic of many ICU patients), this type of constant coverage is not only ideal, it is vitally necessary. As a result, parents of seriously or critically ill children need to be familiar with the hierarchy of an academic hospital, because they will inevitably meet up with a confusing array of doctors in white coats, sometimes individually and at other times when they're traveling in packs.

At the top of the academic medical ladder is the attending physician, also known as "the real doctor." Attending physicians have attended four years of medical school, completed three years of residency, and have completed three more years of subspecialty training. They have completed their entire training, and therefore they answer to no one. They have the final word on a patient's case and are ultimately responsible for the patient. They are also responsible for overall guidance of the medical education team and for coordinating teaching.

These physicians usually participate in research or other scholarly pursuits to satisfy the requirements of the medical school they work for. Depending on their specific title and chosen responsibilities, certain attending physicians devote different amounts of time to the clinical care of patients. As with most people at the top of any organization, attending physicians are the least accessible to others outside the organization. In the case of academic physicians, this means patients and their parents. They usually put in an appearance on morning rounds or afternoon rounds, then retire to virtual seclusion in laboratories or offices. Depending on their accomplishments and publications, academic physicians may be titled assistant professor, associate professor, or, for the most distinguished, professor.

Below the attending physician is the fellow, who is a physician in the midst of a fellowship. Fellowships are training programs in a medical, pediatric, or surgical subspecialty field. These physicians have completed enough training in a standard medicine or pediatric residency to allow them to practice general internal medicine or general pediatrics. They are therefore actually on the same level as one's general pediatrician. Instead of immediately going into practice, however, they have chosen to specialize. Fellows are usually central to both patient care and patient communication in the ICU. Fellows on the medical team know enough and do enough to reliably discuss with parents the current status of a sick child, as well as discuss further plans for and any prognosis of the child. They would bring to the attending physician's attention any problems or issues from staff or parents. As they are still in training, they do not enjoy the privileges of attending physicians, such as ordering what needs to be done from the comfort of office or home or avoiding late-night trips to the hospital when problems develop.

Lower in the academic pecking order, but certainly no less important in terms of actual time spent with patients, are the pediatric residents and interns (interns are first-year residents). One to three years out of medical school, they are the workers in the trenches of any teaching hospital. Residents and interns are called on to draw blood in difficult situations, perform procedures, and initially evaluate patients when problem arise. They are the doctors called on in such situations because they stay overnight in the hospital every third or every fourth night (hence the term *residents*). As they provide the cheap medical labor to staff teaching hospitals around the clock, residents and interns are the most abused and most chronically fatigued members of the team taking care of critically ill children.

These doctors in training are the most visible members of the medical team next to the ICU nurses and can often answer questions from parents regarding issues of daily concern—questions such as, what kind of fluid is dripping through the IV? or is the baby getting fed? or how high was last night's fever and what was it from? or why did so much blood have to be taken that morning? Parents should be prepared for impatient, rushed, or even annoyed responses to their questions, and in my opinion, they should allow for such episodes. After all, these young physicians have either been up for most of the previous night or have to look forward to an incredible amount of work during the rest of that day, or both. They are overworked and underpaid, and they are invariably blamed by parents, superiors, or nurses for any mishap or problem that arises.

Misunderstandings and impatient words are almost guaranteed to occur when professionals such as these are entrusted with the responsibility of answering questions from parents who are themselves extremely stressed by often inconceivable circumstances. Small offenses must be accepted in the proper perspective by all parties involved. Everyone, residents and parents alike, are working for each child's best interests under extremely stressful conditions, often with very little sleep. Residents and interns rarely have enough time to give any individual case a great deal of thought.

Lowest on the academic scale are medical students. One might equate medical students and their role in a teaching hospital with the small flying insects so common in warm weather. These insects generally cause only discomfort as they swarm around and buzz annoyingly. Other than causing a lot of extra work as we try to avoid or exterminate them, they seem to serve no purpose. Were it not for these insignificant little bugs, however, the entire food chain would fall apart. Larger insects would starve without their smaller prey, thus depriving birds and mammals of their food. Ultimately larger, more important animals would eventually become affected.

Such is the fate of medical students, who seem only to add more work to their supervising doctors without actually reducing anyone's workload or directly helping patients. They actually pay large amounts of money for the opportunity to learn medicine while being abused, overworked, and sometimes simply ignored by residents or attending physicians simply too busy to always teach. Without medical students, however, the future of medicine would be dismal, as would be the future of medical progress through research and teaching.

Parents should be very cautious about relying on answers and opinions from medical students, especially regarding sensitive or prognostic issues. Medical students' egos tend to be inflated under the best of circumstances, especially if they are mistaken for actual doctors by unwitting parents taken in by their white coats. This cautionary view is drawn from my own mistakes as a medical student, as opposed to anything that may have occurred during Andrew's time in the hospital. At the time, I was justifiably reproached by my supervising resident for spewing out all sorts of facts and opinions in response to a parent's questions about her child. My answers were wrong and misleading. But her trust in me, or in what my white coat and stethoscope represented, proved too tempting a compliment to resist. As a resident and later an attending physician, I have witnessed similar behavior from the students I supervised. It is an easy trap to fall into as a medical student eager to impress—and a trap parents should at least be aware of.

One of the most common complaints of parents caught up in the turmoil of a teaching hospital is the difficulty in keeping all the people in white coats straight. Instead of the trusted family doctor coming by each day to give his or her opinion, parents may be suddenly besieged by a large group of people attired in white coats, usually conversing among themselves in an unintelligible language. Appearance alone doesn't necessarily help sort them out. A semblance of knowledge about one's case also may not single out the responsible white-coated caregiver a parent should turn to. Doctors (3) from medical students up to fellows may be willing to share information or opinions about the patients they are involved with.

Typically, the entire team will make rounds together and visit each patient in the morning. The attending physician and fellow will stand out by their leadership demeanor and impressive lecturing to the group. Academic ICUs are usually closed to parents and family during morning round times, however, to allow rounds to proceed efficiently. However, parents and patients should realize that anyone on the academic physician team responsible for a patient may offer some information, or at least relay questions or concerns to higher-ups to address. For issues of great concern, such as prognosis, implications of a test, the specific test results themselves, and the timing of important interventions such as weaning a patient from a ventilator, parents should not be shy about asking specifically for the fellow overseeing their child's case. Chances are the attending physician probably won't be available, and the fellow probably knows more about the individual case anyway.

In my opinion, parents should make it their business to know which white coat is in charge and has the best idea of the overall case. Important information should be obtained from that physician. Information obtained by caregivers who may be more immediately accessible may be helpful and certainly well intentioned. If delivered from a junior member, though, that information or opinion could be incomplete or could be given without a clear view of the entire case. A parent doesn't need confusion to be added to the stress and uncertainty they are already embroiled in.

Categorizing members of the team taking care of one's child is only the beginning of understanding the world of academic medicine. Placing the role of academic medicine as a whole into the proper perspective with regard to the actual patients it serves is much more difficult. In any profession, a practitioner becomes skilled through repeated hands-on experience under the supervision of more experienced colleagues. From the retail clerk to the police officer responding to an alarm to the teacher responsible for a child's education, no one could carry out responsibilities successfully by simply reading about the job first and then jumping in unsupervised. Certainly the same should apply to the practitioner responsible for one's very health. The problem lies in finding the appropriate balance between passing on knowledge and providing care to patients. Emphasis on maintaining educational excellence may result in a critically ill child dispassionately treated as a tool of learning, although the child may admittedly be receiving very good medical treatment. Is the assurance of excellent care, delivered by the most learned specialists in the area, worth the atmosphere of detached, sometimes self-serving emphasis on education-preoccupied caregivers?

Certainly the opportunities for learning about medicine are most plentiful among patients hospitalized in the ICU. In that precarious setting, the entire spectrum of human physiology and pathology is on display, technology abounds, and intricate procedures are always available to perform and subsequently learn about. And in that setting, emotions run high among parents and other family members. In such a pressurized atmosphere, do medical science and compassionate caregiving conflict or complement? Some may feel it makes no difference; the two worlds will coexist regardless of personal preference and will need to be tolerated when a child requires the care that only specialized academic institutions can provide. I do not mean to imply that such care is always cold and impersonal, either. Physicians such as Dr. R are certainly present in all medical schools. Unfortunately, though, the emphasis by many physicians in the midst of their training can easily shift toward gaining knowledge and impressing superiors. The key to reconciling possible conflict and misunderstanding between academicians and civilians rests on the academicians. I believe doctors are responsible for emphasizing to their charges that compassion and dignity are qualities every bit as important as knowledge and insight into complex illness. Teaching must be done, and it must involve patients themselves. Physicians must teach at the bedside as if they themselves were in the bed, staring up into the intimidating faces of white-clad strangers almost leering back in undisguised fascination.

Sometimes, however, even the most well-meaning attempt at compassionately pointing out physical findings or at lecturing on why a particular child is so interesting may prove too painful for a parent to tolerate. A parent should always reserve the right to ask if teaching or demonstration of bedside findings could be performed later. It is indeed true that the standard admitting form patients or their parents sign upon admission to a teaching hospital typically includes consent for physicians-in-training to administer care to patients.

As both a former academic physician and as the parent of a Great Teaching Case, I firmly believe that the right to consolation and compassion supersedes the right or duty to enhance medical education. Such consideration does not necessarily contradict the terms of the admission contract, nor does it represent any serious set back to the hallowed institution of academic teaching. There will always be other opportunities for teaching under more acceptable conditions, and there will always be many other Great Cases waiting for their findings to come under the spotlight of inquiring doctors. Delaying a round of bedside instruction may very well avoid generating mistrust and resentment over intrusive interactions, emotions difficult to defuse once ignited. There may not be many more opportunities, however, for parents to console and comfort a critically ill or terminally ill child already frightened by illness and by the hospital environment.

Chapter 3

Ethical Considerations

We finally came back home to stay after our visit to Dr. S in New York. Now that Ruth and I were more assured of our son's diagnosis, as bad as it was, we could get down to the business of resuming our lives and confronting all the sad little details of a life with such a child. First, we had to make sure he would never suffer needlessly. That meant we had to clarify what should and would be done for Andrew when he started to fail, as we were told he inevitably would. We had witnessed firsthand what was done for (or to) many dying patients, both adults and children. The tubes and needle sticks that invaded patients' bodies, and the pain, discomfort, and indignities that were committed in the name of prolonging life for a few more arduous undignified days or weeks, brutalized my thoughts as I considered that inevitable future.

We first met with the pediatric ethicist, who was also a well-respected pediatric cancer specialist, at the hospital to review all the legal and ethical implications of our situation. As a physician who had to help families almost daily deal with dying relatives during my rotations in the intensive care unit (ICU), I had always looked with disdain on medical ethicists. I thought such physicians prattled on about the many philosophical ways a particular heart-wrenching situation could be viewed. They could discuss at length the could be's, or they would play devil's advocate when considering any complex ethical problem—always as interested third parties but never getting their hands dirty or enduring the consequences of a decision. Accordingly, I was less than enthusiastic about meeting with such a doctor about my own child.

I reluctantly went along with Ruth and was pleasantly surprised at the medical ethicist's candor and nonjudgmental advice. He assured us that if there were truly no hope for Andrew's long-term survival, we were not obligated as parents to provide anything that would uselessly prolong life. This meant avoiding intubation, intravenous or oral medications, or other medical interventions. He also advised that we were not obligated to provide even basic life support, such as artificial nutrition through veins or tubes, if Andrew became unable to take in enough food on his own. After hearing all the uproar in the news about families prevented from removing tube feedings from brain-damaged relatives, I felt distinctly uncomfortable even thinking about doing such a thing to my own baby.

In our case, however, this doctor claimed that placing Andrew on artificial support of any kind, including even nutrition and hydration, was inappropriate since he had a terminal progressive illness. Of course, the decision remained a very individual one, and such a decision may not be the same for parents who may believe that absolute preservation of life, instead of quality of life, should be the ultimate goal. We could medicate our son to spare him pain and discomfort, and we could hold him when the end was near, but we were not forced to have doctors place tubes or intravenous lines.

This specialist altered my perception of what a detached third party could offer to a personal and difficult discussion. My cynical view was softened, but not totally changed. Looking back, it was probably this doctor's open, honest, and direct demeanor that impressed me the most. He never shied away from giving us what we so desperately sought: an honest, helpful opinion. He certainly didn't put us off with false hope, not when bluntly confronting only how best to comfort and console a dying child. He could have danced around the issue and turned our questions back to us, sounding quite important but not really providing us with anything substantial. He was truly a credit to his profession.

I had walked out of each successive talk we'd had about Andrew thinking that it would be the saddest experience I would ever have to endure. And yet, from that first conversation with Dr. R to the Boston specialist to the current somber discussion with this ethicist, the finality and bleakness seemed to get worse. We weren't talking about how to cope with the sad obligation of having to send our child to day care, or how tragic it was going to be when Ruth had to return to work instead of remaining a full-time mother. Ruth and I were seeking counsel on how to make our baby's death as painless and as dignified as possible.

Like our experiences with Dr. R and Dr. S, the advice of this ethicist nonetheless gave us some degree of bittersweet consolation despite the actual topic. I had previously envisioned Ruth and me at the center of legal and social turmoil when the public found out how two doctors had wanted their baby to die instead of caring for him and doing everything for him to the bitter end. We were acutely aware of the "Baby Doe" ruling, which had recently been publicized. This court decision mandated that hospital workers or even family members should alert the state if a baby or child were being deprived of necessary care or sustenance regardless of condition, illness, or prognosis. The assurances of this doctor, then, relieved to a large degree my constant paranoia over spies among the hospital staff who would report our intentions to the state. I had actually imagined the newspaper headlines about us: "Parents Prevented from Starving Baby to Death by State Intervention." So many years later, it all sounds egocentric and overblown, but at the time, we were anything but clear-headed. And the Baby Doe ruling was real and intended to be enforced. In the end, we remained horribly saddened but at least at peace with the necessity and the permission to treat our son in what we considered was a loving and humane way, without fearing invasion from uninvolved strangers.

The final step entailed meeting with our pediatrician and enacting what we had discussed formally and legally. As with everything else we had endured through Andrew's brief life, I was now experiencing personally a hardship I had previously supervised as a physician. We met with Andrew's pediatrician and her associate after office hours one evening. Our talk was honest and surprisingly supportive. We stated that all we wanted was to let nature take its course without causing unnecessary pain or suffering. No hospitalization, no intravenous medicines or oxygen tents, no artificial feedings. It was not a course of action some, perhaps many, people would understand, but it was one that Ruth and I felt very strongly about. Andrew's pediatrician was supportive; she promised to do everything possible to look out for Andrew's comfort. This was the same physician who had left no stone unturned, who had personally found repeated second opinions for us and had done everything possible to preserve Andrew's life. Now she was putting forth the same dedication to provide comfort to his life as much as possible.

She documented in Andrew's chart all that we had agreed on. After tears and hugs, we left, our belief and trust in the medical establishment to a large degree restored. We left feeling overwhelmingly sad, but just as important, we left at peace with what had been decided. Possibly when the moment of truth actually arrived we would feel differently. Until then, we had been unable to help Andrew at all, other than to drag him from one specialist to another. That feeling of helplessness was almost as difficult to bear as was the sadness. We not only gained a sense of peace from our visit with our pediatrician, but we also erased that disheartening feeling of helplessness. It was a pathetic triumph—to finally help our son by assuring he would be spared from discomfort for as long as he lived.

And so we finished planning for Andrew's future. To the usual couple, planning a child's future would conjure up visions of putting money aside for college, collecting savings bonds, and storing up all of one's own childhood toys for their child's eventual use. "Planning for Andrew's future" meant carefully planning out the details of his premature death and trying to avoid anything that could cause any more emotional or physical pain. Something was definitely wrong with this picture. The usually optimistic hope of a parent for a child had twisted into a dark countdown toward finality. There may have been peace, but pain certainly conquered everything.

From a purely selfish point of view, assuring my child's quality of life, however short that life was, eased whatever doubts I may have carried about the convictions I had expressed to my patients. Slow, lingering death was an all-too-common result of hospitalization in the hospital's ICU. As the physician on service in that ICU, I had counseled many families about letting go and allowing nature to take its course without subjecting their loved one to futile medical intervention. I had always felt just a little guilty inside, thinking how easy it was to give such advice when I was the personally uninvolved, professional physician, wondering deep inside if I would accept such advice if things were reversed.

Now things *were* reversed, and I had at least remained true to my convictions. Every person has his own convictions about what constitutes a life worth living. Some of my current patients choose to be supported by a ventilator, sometimes unable to move at all. Others choose to live only as long as artificial support can be avoided. Such issues are not matters of absolute right or absolute wrong. What would qualify as only existing for some would truly be living for others. Ruth and I had had the benefit, if such a euphemistic word can be used, of facing down this issue from without and from within. We had seen how modern medicine could intervene and prolong life. With little uncertainty, we had chosen to let our child live without such invasion, not to simply exist with it.

The Golden Rule

A comprehensive discussion of ethical decisions, especially as they apply to children, is far beyond the scope of my professional expertise and of this book. In fact, because of the complexity and the inherently individual nature of such issues, no single generic text can do justice to this topic. My professional and personal experiences can, however, shed some light onto the agonizing decisions parents may have to face regarding their child's future.

As a pulmonologist who treats adult patients, my duties have often included overseeing all aspects of a medical ICU. My presenting patients and families with difficult ethical dilemmas and harsh truths has become an unfortunately common responsibility, occurring sometimes daily. During the first two years of my son's life, and to a lesser extent later on, I needed to confront similar difficult ethical issues born out of the possibility of Andrew's severe disability and premature death.

Even such professional and personal experience does not make the advice or judgments in this book universally valid or truthful. The only absolute judgment my experiences entitle me to declare with any certainty is that there never should be one absolute judgment or truth when considering serious illness. Each situation is individual and different, and deserves consideration on a family-by-family and child-by-child basis. This is the Golden Rule of ethics; I have arrived at it from living through both sides of an issue rarely even considered by most parents, much less endured.

Meaningful quality of life or *unacceptable suffering* are phrases that mean different things to different people. Very rarely is there an absolute wrong way to view hopeless or terminal illness. Whether social worker, physician, or member of the clergy, there is no room for blanket judgments on what constitutes an acceptable quality of life. This doesn't mean, however, that decisions regarding dying or suffering children should be left to parents without concerned outside opinions and information. Many physicians feel, with the best and most compassionate of intentions, that they are merely staying within the deeply personal nature of ethical decisions by only presenting the medical implications of each possible course of action without giving their own advice or direction. I progressed through medical training with the same belief, knowing I was doing the right thing by preserving the patient's and family's right to a private and personal decision. Only after years of practice and many discussions with patients and their families did I come to doubt the correctness of this approach. I found that by trying not to intrude or invade a family's right to a private decision, I was essentially offering them a virtual Chinese menu of ethical decisions. I left them free to mix and match all possible ethical resolutions to each complex medical issue that arose to be confronted. This approach certainly preserved privacy and individuality, but often it did so at the price of confusion and profound guilt over the difficult choices to be made. Ultimately, I came to feel that I was abdicating part of my responsibility as their physician.

Most ethical decisions concerning the care and comfort of terminally ill or critically ill patients are necessarily based on complicated medical probabilities and elaborate physiology. As such, the opinion and input of a physician cognizant of both the individual circumstances and of the scientific facts as they relate to those circumstances is crucial to any decision made. No doctor would give parents choices of different antibiotics and expect the parents to choose between them for their child. Although the gravity and complexity of ethical decisions to be made for a child obviously differ in scope from the more tangible choice of antibiotic, informed medical guidance remains an appropriate need.

So what guidance can I as a physician and suffering parent offer to other parents facing unimaginable decisions for their sick children? First, I would hope that the description of our thoughts as we attempted to comprehend and then confront the news that our child was going to die a slow but inevitable death will at least provide one small measure of comfort: no matter how unthinkable or difficult the decisions about one's child become, they have been suffered through by other parents before. Second, I intend these words to provide some sense of empowerment for parents embroiled in these overwhelming circumstances. Parents have the right to do what they consider right for their children without fearing judgment from uninvolved professionals, ethicists, or civilians who would not have to endure the direct consequences of their opinions. The Golden Rule trumps any opinions of absolute, whether well intentioned or not. Finally, modern medical practice often does not allow adequate time or resources to appropriately guide parents and families through the ethical and legal intricacies of critically ill and terminally ill children. My experiences are relayed from a position of inside knowledge and power, but they are also relayed from a position of helplessness and grief. I hope that the words and thoughts I have chronicled here will support the thoughts and doubts of other parents facing similar circumstances as they try to answer questions that may be too frightening to even be broached by responsible parties.

These issues are certain to become more common as the technology that drives modern medicine continues to advance. Witness the cases of families and parents prevented, or at least prosecuted, for removing children from life support. Some of those children have been young adults who have been vegetative for years. More rarely, instances have involved young children or infants. Many of these cases share in common the intervention of outside parties into the intensely personal emotions and decisions forced on parents by critical or terminal illness. Such well-intentioned attempts to protect the best interests of a child may result only in sharpening the agony and turmoil already affecting all those personally involved.

The notion of doing what is in the best interest of the child does not always equate to life at any cost. A child's best interest should not be dogmatically interpreted. Opinions of outside, dispassionate professionals may be useful in establishing general ethical guidelines and in defining legal boundaries, but responsibility can only rest with those relatives and doctors intimately involved and thus ultimately accountable. Only by openly acknowledging all sides and options when confronting a child's serious illness will the hysteria and needless additional anxiety be reduced.

The Realities of a Terminally Ill Child

Ruth and I finally settled in with Andrew at home, intending never to see the inside of a hospital or listen to another specialist again as long as possible. We'd expected to have come home with a new baby several months, and a couple of lifetimes, earlier. Everything that only happens to other people had actually happened to us, and now we had arrived home, ready to pick up the pieces.

A routine at home was surprisingly easy to get back into. After all, having our terminally ill baby near us all the time was certainly easier than going back and forth to a hospital, as we had been doing since Andrew was born. Certain rearrangement needed attending to, however, to accommodate our circumstances. We had been warned that as a terminally ill infant with a neuromuscular disease (it was still wrenchingly difficult to truly comprehend that as our reality), Andrew could die literally at any time. That meant he could never sleep in his brother's room, as we had intended; Daniel might otherwise become an unexpected witness to his brother's death, possibly while the rest of us were asleep. It was a lot for any relative to bear—and far too horrible to contemplate happening to Andrew's four-year-old brother. So we dismantled the crib and took it instead into our bedroom. Several months earlier, setting up that crib had been a blissful chore, as it had represented the new hopes and dreams we had for the new baby. Now I was setting it up to provide a quiet, private place for a baby to die, close to us so that we would be immediately aware when he started to choke or struggle to breathe.

The feeding tube in Andrew's nose was not as easily dealt with. It was necessary because he was simply too weak to be able to take in enough nutrition on his own, as we had demonstrated time and again during his hospitalization. He would take his usual two or so ounces of formula at each feeding before becoming exhausted, after which we would pour the remainder into a bag. The bag would be attached to the feeding tube, and we would then spend the next ten minutes trying to out-think the pump that regulated the flow of formula out of that bag and into Andrew.

I had walked past such pumps in the hospital every day on rounds without ever giving them a second thought. I had catheterized hearts and had figured out complex metabolic illnesses, but I could not master programming that damn pump without several tries. I couldn't imagine how other parents managed suction catheters, urinary catheters, and respirators for their children. Even getting the pump to work each time gave me little satisfaction, since feeding my baby through a plastic tube was not my idea of father and son tenderly bonding while feeding.

After the first several days home, it was time to change the feeding tube. Andrew had been picking at the bandages holding it in place, wrinkling his nose at the discomfort it caused, and crying frequently. The tube caused us a great deal of discomfort as well, since it really was the only visible reminder that Andrew was anything other than a normal baby. Although not as obscenely disruptive as a tracheostomy tube, the thin feeding tube still prevented us from looking beyond Andrew as a child with a disability and focusing on Andrew as just our new baby. Changing the tube was a terrible experience. He writhed as we pulled the old tube out through his nose; then he gagged and cried as we inserted another into his nose and forced it into his esophagus. I would have gladly volunteered to take his place many times over; nothing would have been more painful than inflicting such brutality on my own son.

It may seem like a relatively small matter, given everything else we and Andrew had been subjected to, as the tube itself was quite thin and was inserted into an opening that was already there. Balanced against causing Andrew such discomfort by inserting it, however, was the fact that without it Andrew could not eat enough on his own to survive. The possibility of inflicting that tube change on Andrew time after time made us confront an agonizing choice: should we continue putting Andrew through the pain and discomfort we had just gone to such lengths to protect him from, or should we pull the tube for good, let him take in what he could, and watch him slowly starve to death? Once we dared even raise such questions, more doubts and emotions were unleashed. Were we really considering stopping the tube feedings out of concern for Andrew's comfort, or did Ruth and I fear that painful ritual and the realization that he was far less than perfect? Would Andrew ever forgive us for starving him? Would we ever forgive ourselves? Never would I have believed one simple act could have provoked such turmoil. The more we considered it, the greater the implications of our indecision became. Do we keep prolonging suffering (his or ours?) by preserving life, or do we hasten our son's death through starvation?

We delayed making our decision another week, until it came time to change that tube again, but the time did of course arrive. As we held Andrew the night before, it struck us that if we could do nothing else, we could hold him and protect him from discomfort. I don't know why it seemed so much clearer to us that night. Nothing special had occurred to grant us such a revelation. Nonetheless, we both felt very comfortable with our decision to not replace the feeding tube but instead to let nature take its course, as it would eventually do anyway, and to dedicate ourselves to making the inevitable happen as compassionately as possible. The next day, I was acutely aware of the meaning behind our action. Pulling out the feeding tube would only take a minute, yet it would affect us for a lifetime. After Andrew had finished crying, Ruth and I picked him up and held him again. For the first time since his bout with pneumonia, we were actually able to see and caress his entire face without bandages or tubes violating it. Just that small change, easy to take for granted under other circumstances, was enough of a gift to firm our resolve.

Just like most other events that had shaped Andrew's short life so far, however, things did not work out as expected. Andrew somehow, inexplicably, did not go on to succumb, as every specialist and every test had warned us he would. He actually began to take more formula on his own. If fed frequently enough, it seemed as if he was able to take in enough nutrition to sustain himself. "Miraculous" may perhaps be too dramatic a word to describe what happened after the tube was pulled out. But after preparing ourselves for a child's certain death from starvation and dehydration, it seemed about the only word to explain what we were seeing. Each day, Andrew continued to take in increasing amounts of formula until Ruth and I were convinced that the future might be a little more hopeful after all. It wouldn't be the last time Andrew defeated the predictions and diagnoses of the medical establishment. We couldn't explain why Andrew was suddenly able to eat and drink enough to sustain his life, but explaining it didn't seem nearly as important as living it. Besides, by then, we had given up trying to explain anything.

Our lives gradually regained a little more balance. The excitement that fills the houses of most newborns was of course gone, but the little tasks of feeding Andrew, rocking and holding him, and giving him baths could now be enjoyed. Our two other children doted on Andrew as well. Our six-year-old was anxious to hold and feed Andrew despite Andrew's frailty, and even our four-year-old son tried playing with him. Andrew himself would occasionally smile at us. Life in our household approached something close to normal. Each time we picked Andrew up, though, Ruth and I noticed that although Andrew may not have dehydrated and failed, he remained weak and fragile. Any unsupported area or extremity hung limply, unable to move the least little bit against gravity. What he lacked in strength, however, Andrew made up for in personality. He remained bright, alert, and interactive, and he smiled more each passing day.

The anguish we had suffered in our discussions about Andrew's comfort care, followed by what we had thought would be the finality of our decision to remove the feeding tube, gradually ebbed. We were left with a dull ache, like the constant throb that lingers after the initial searing pain of a burn starts to fade. We were grateful for Andrew's inexplicable survival without tube feedings, but the big picture unfortunately hadn't changed. We simply tried to move on while bracing ourselves for the inevitable.

It is an issue that any reasonable parent would have difficulty thinking about, much less experiencing. But preparing for the future of a child who has been denied a future is an unfortunate reality that some parents must face, often with little knowledge of where to begin or what to expect. Our personal experiences with defining and confronting Andrew's terminal illness demonstrate the reality of this situation. Our discussions with the physicians involved in Andrew's case, and our subsequent decisions, exemplify how parents and the medical establishment can work together and make a terrible situation more tolerable and humane. Our experiences were not all that different from what others in similar circumstances might experience, even though Ruth and I were treated more as fellow physicians than as agonized parents. We certainly hadn't been treated all that deferentially. I believe Andrew's physicians had dealt just as compassionately with other patients' parents not associated with the medical field.

The key, then, is not hoping that you as parents have certain qualities or have a position that entitles you to particular consideration. The key is to find doctors who recognize how exceptional such a situation is and who will do all they can to treat you accordingly. "Honest communication" may sound trite and insincere, but we found it to be a major weapon against the crushing distress that can destroy a family trying to cope with a seriously ill or terminally ill child. Parents should not be hesitant to confront their child's physician about what the future holds, nor should they be afraid to voice expectations or doubts about what is being done or what should be done.

These views, born of our own personal experience, are actually supported by recent peer-reviewed medical literature. Studies and scientific discussions about terminal care are increasingly being published in well-respected journals. Such a push has been fostered by Oregon's legalization of physician-assisted suicide, by Jack Kevorkian's actions and subsequent conviction, and by the swelling ranks of seriously ill patients surviving longer and more precariously. One of many important articles reached a surprisingly candid conclusion. A study of the economic and emotional burdens of providing care to adults with terminal illness was published in *Annals of Internal Medicine* (March 21, 2000; 132:451–459). The authors concluded that of all the factors leading to stress and hardship for caregivers, few could really be meaningfully changed or improved upon. Only one intervention seemed to make a difference: "Caregivers of patients...who reported that the physicians they dealt with listened to their needs and opinions...were significantly less likely to be depressed than caregivers who dealt with physicians who did not listen."(p. 458). Furthermore, the study suggested "that empathetic physicians who listen to patients and caregivers can reduce some of the burdens on caregivers (and their depression)."(p. 458). Certainly more dispassionate studies and discerning articles can be expected to appear in the medical literature. The topic of communication and compassion is not as amenable to statistical evaluation and impartial review as disease processes or controlled trials of medications. Yet each attempt to confront it in scientific journals lends more credibility to the intangible side of medicine I defend as remaining so important.

Because each case of a critically or terminally ill child is obviously individual, addressing specific concerns about certain diseases or reaching particular ethical decisions would be inappropriate here. After all, the Golden Rule should always be the most important consideration. Every situation, every sick child, every set of parents trying to confront the circumstances that they have been thrown into, deserve individual concern, without any blanketing right-or-wrong judgments. My own experience demonstrates how difficult it is for everyone involved to arrive at "the right thing" for a terminally ill child and how easy it becomes to succumb to real doubts and imagined pressures.

I can also address specific realities of terminal illness once parents have resolved themselves to a course of action or comfort. First and foremost, a decision against heroic or life-sustaining intervention must be carefully documented in the medical record. The medical record only goes so far, however. It does provide after-the-fact, indisputable documentation of previous actions and discussions. In reality, though, it is usually not immediately available in the event of unforeseen occurrences or at the time of a predicted but still disturbing catastrophe. Written documentation may therefore best serve to reinforce and strengthen parents' resolve to enact their decisions at the moment of truth, regardless of how such instructions may be perceived. Arguments by other health care professionals who become involved at the time of crisis may be understandably born out of a well-meaning desire to do everything possible for a sick child. Life-prolonging and uncomfortable acts of resuscitation may occur during the confusion and anxiety of a medical crisis unless parents are present and are able to voice what they had determined and documented to be in their child's best interests. Frenzied last-minute interventions do happen.

Our attempt to convey our wishes to caregivers illustrates these complexities. We needed to inform our visiting nurses of Andrew's status, since one of them could very well be the only one at home with Andrew in the event of a sudden setback. We believed at that time that Andrew would live at most for two years and would only become more disabled before finally succumbing. As doctors and as parents, we knew that Andrew would do nothing but suffer needlessly once placed on a ventilator during resuscitation. Accordingly, our wishes for Andrew had been clearly spelled out. Supported with this documentation, we asked the nurses that if Andrew should start to choke or have trouble breathing, we should be called immediately instead of 911. We further asked that he be simply hugged and soothed until we arrived home. If he were to die before we were able to make it home, at least we would know he had been comfortable.

The association governing the visiting nurses refused to comply with our wishes. They did acknowledge the reality of Andrew's terminal disease. Nonetheless, they insisted on calling rescue in the event of any problems, no matter how much we assured them that their only responsibility was to make Andrew comfortable in our absence. The discussion itself was painful enough; arguing over how best to allow our child to die was excruciating. We chose not to pursue respite at home through standard home care channels and finally found appropriate care through a hospice organization.

Reality cannot be changed or avoided by following dogmatic beliefs and imposing such ideals on others. The decision Ruth and I made is certainly not the only ethical decision to be reached in such a situation. Other parents would justifiably feel more comfortable preserving a child's life at any cost, and we have known parents who have done just that, without regrets. Both quality and quantity of life are important considerations, although judgments regarding quality of life are necessarily more subjective. There is no moral high ground of absolute right or wrong; there is only that which parents determine is in the best interest of a child who they love and only want the best for. It has become clear to me, on the basis of episodes such as the one I just described, that continued attention by parents to this most important of issues remains necessary despite documentation in the medical record.

That said, I would still caution how easy it is to self-righteously violate the Golden Rule. Now able to look back more objectively, I realize that I had been unable to accept that anyone could view quality of life in any other way than what we had chosen for Andrew. At the time, Ruth and I became almost enraged at even the suggestion that artificially prolonging life for someone with Andrew's prognosis would be a reasonable alternative to consider. It was certainly a presumptuous violation of my own Golden Rule. Since then, I have known members of several families who have indeed chosen such an alternative path.

One family in particular stands out in my mind. The family comprised a mother and her son. Through the cruel course of muscular dystrophy, her son had slowly progressed over the years to almost total immobility, eventually becoming unable to breathe on his own. A permanent tracheostomy was placed, allowing him to depend on a ventilator at all times. He communicated through eye movements and by mouthing words. For literally decades, these two had drawn strength from each other, lived with and depended on each other, and had come to accept the ventilator, the constant suctioning, the recurrent infections, and the hospitalizations as small prices to pay for allowing them to continue living together. I was the attending physician during the son's last admission. He finally succumbed to overwhelming pneumonia. His mother had nothing but good memories of their last twenty or so years together, and apparently her son had felt the same satisfaction. They had lived, not simply existed or endured.

Another similar family taught me similar lessons. They lived in a small town in northern Missouri, where technology and innovation was much more commonly associated with farm machinery as opposed to medical care. The son had slowly progressive Duchenne muscular dystrophy, similar to the previous family. He had also progressed to almost total immobility by the time he presented to my clinic, but did not require the use of a tracheostomy and mechanical ventilation. This twenty-one year old man followed high school, college, and professional sports avidly, kept in touch with others through his computer, and seemed to be accepted in this small rural community without bias. He rode through heart failure, progressive breathing difficulty, and frightening episodes of lung infection with calm acceptance and determination. His parents were similarly courageous. They came to each clinic visit with questions and concerns, but never demanded, never spent time bemoaning misfortune. They carefully looked into options for their son on both the Internet and through my services, but spent equal time making sure their son enjoyed activities in which any young person would participate.

He died suddenly while cheering for his team at a basketball game. At his funeral, everyone spoke of his hobbies and contributions; his illness was only alluded to, not focused on. His friends and family weren't covering up or hiding his illness. His disability had simply not prevented satisfaction with life or enjoyment of friends and family, and was apparently not going to become the focus after he died.

I have had the honor of serving other families caught up in similar circumstances in my capacity as a pulmonologist: mother and son facing years of the son's quadriplegia; a family rising above the complete immobility and ventilator dependence of a woman's amyotrophic lateral sclerosis (known as ALS and sometimes called Lou Gehrig disease). I have met parents who felt fulfilled as they cared for children with severe physical disabilities or with severe cognitive impairment. Quality of life was certainly different for those families, but it was satisfying for them all. In fact, watching firsthand how those families overcame such obstacles and how some parents and children live through them and accept their lifestyle as meaningful and complete, has in turn provided me a great deal of unexpected gratification as a physician and parent.

So I have come to accept that a future deemed unimaginable for me and my family may not be indisputably agreed upon by others facing similar difficulties. My experiences as a physician have entitled me to insights into the details and the wearisome and uncomfortable responsibilities thrust upon parents and families as a result of artificially prolonging life. These insights do not automatically imbue me or any physician or outside party with the authority to judge right or wrong for others. I offer guidelines for parents facing difficult situations that are based on years of medical practice. It is not intended to unequivocally support my own philosophy as the right one. I lost sight of the Golden Rule amidst the maelstrom of Andrew's illness. I have subsequently learned that in the world of overwhelming medical tragedy, it is never too late to learn from others, and it is never too difficult to become more tolerant of different philosophies.

These lessons have indeed entered the medical literature as well. Satisfaction with quality of life has been found to be surprisingly high among patients and families who have chosen to sustain life by mechanical ventilation and other such intensive support. One such study surveyed patients with Duchenne muscular dystrophy who had elected ventilator support (Duchenne muscular dystrophy is the most common type of muscular dystrophy, and eventually results in death from respiratory or heart failure. Andrew has congenital muscular dystrophy, a different muscle disease with a different prognosis). The majority of these patients contacted were satisfied with their lives, and very satisfied with their family life (Bach JR, et al. Life satisfaction of individuals with Duchenne muscular dystrophy using long-term mechanical ventilatory support. *American Journal of Physical Medicine & Rehabilitation* 1991 June 70:129-135).

Another study (Oppenheimer EA. Decision-making in the respiratory care of amyotrophic lateral sclerosis: should home mechanical ventilation be used? *Palliative Care* 1993 7(suppl 2):49-64) confirmed this attitude among patients with amyotrophic lateral sclerosis (ALS). Further, *both* studies found that health care professionals tend to significantly underestimate such patients' fulfillment and satisfaction with life, which may then affect counseling and advice on life sustaining therapies.

It should be remembered that all the patients in these studies were adults, not infants or children. It is difficult to know how to generalize these conclusions to children Andrew's age. I still view these studies as admirable attempts to confront the most difficult and personal issues that patients and families must face. I also feel they provide support for my Golden Rule.

Two final caveats remain when determining appropriate action for an extremely ill child. First, even when a decision is made and put down in writing in a formal legal document such as a patient chart, it is not irreversible. The people legally responsible for someone's health care, whether it is for one's self, for a child, or for an adult relative who can no longer act for themselves, always have the ability and right to change a decision they made previously. People always retain the right to change their minds, sometimes not until the last minute. Advance directives are designed to give peace of mind, not to forever limit care to a directive that was decided under different circumstances or in a different frame of mind.

The last caveat about terminal illness, which I have learned as both a parent and physician: the certainty of a terminal prognosis as rendered by the best of modern medical wisdom and delivered with conviction is not always certain. Usually this is the case; but not always. I have seen Andrew defeat several "certain" life expectancies and become a child who outlived hospice care. As a physician, I have personally managed patients who continue to survive and persevere through certain terminal illness. My favorite case is that of a woman who presented with overwhelming respiratory failure, which itself should have killed her. She also suffered severe brain damage from low oxygen during that hospitalization, which also should have killed her. She has subsequently recovered from severe heart failure and severe pneumonia, any one of which should have killed her. And she did this all in the face of suffering from ALS, which itself is a terminal disease. Yet she continues to offer me an astonishing education to this day, years after her diagnosis. She is on a ventilator and immobile, but she is alive and full of life.

Are these exceptions? Absolutely. They nonetheless have taught me, more than any book or class, that in some circumstances labeled terminal or hopeless there can be room for hope. It must be counseled responsibly, because nothing is more cruel than succumbing to the temptation of false hope. Usually only time can reveal room for hope; compassion provides the support, no matter what the passage of time brings.

Siblings and the Realities of the Terminally or Chronically Ill Child

Very worthwhile organizations such as Hospice have become available to help a family cope with chronically or terminally ill family members. However, getting through severe illness or even death must go beyond professional outside support and must depend on the family itself. With this particular issue, my insights into family dynamics aren't really made any more valuable by wearing the white coat instead of relying on it. Each family is unique. Thus, for better or for worse, parents will learn how best to help their families cope through their own personal experience, if such unfortunate circumstances must be confronted at all. Our family's journey through Andrew's illness may offer other parents an understanding of how to attend to the health and outcome of the critically ill child's siblings.

Ever since we learned of Andrew's prognosis, we had resolved to be honest with Andrew's brother and sister. At the time of his birth, Emily was six years old, and Daniel was four and a half years old. Much of our resolve was based on our belief in the inevitability of Andrew's death. We were faced with the need to somehow strike a balance between assuring that Emily and Daniel would get to know and appreciate a new brother, as they should, but at the same time teaching them about the realities of illness and death and how both were going to have their brother taken away. We honestly weren't sure the latter aspect of that responsibility was even appropriate for such young children. Why not just let Emily and Daniel enjoy their brother while they could, just as all their friends were able to do with their own newborn siblings? The ugliness of sickness, disability, and death could follow at some point, perhaps when they were older and better able to understand it.

Putting off the truth was tempting for several reasons. Ruth and I certainly didn't need to add any more stress to our lives. Dealing with one child's critical illness, then trying to accept a terminal outlook, drained us as it was. Selfishly, we could at least come home and have hopes for the future somewhat restored by Emily's and Daniel's normal enjoyment of life. And for Emily and Daniel themselves, why not preserve their childhoods for as long as possible? They'd have years to learn and experience the darker side of life. Why not learn about it in easier-to-handle small bits over years, and let them just be children for now? But no matter how tempting the preservation of their innocence looked, and no matter how inviting the preservation of our own emotional stability seemed, Andrew's condition was affecting us and had undoubtedly been intruding into his siblings' lives as well. Andrew's illness was happening, and his death was going to happen. We realized that there isn't *any* time in a child's life that is a particularly better time to deal with a sibling's death, whether they are five, ten, or fifteen. Even a younger child could probably understand and confront such a terrible event when gently but openly prepared for it. Further, Andrew's illness was serious but certainly not shameful, and we were worried that to Emily and Daniel, it might appear that we were covering up Andrew's illness because we were ashamed of him. Childhood innocence and a family's stability cannot be preserved by delaying, sparing, or sugar-coating the pain of reality. Not even the kindest and most compassionate of good intentions can change reality. The goal should rather be to give as much support as possible to brothers and sisters, to demonstrate by actions and words that sadness is natural, and to allow the siblings to share in the caring for the affected sibling and to experience the day-to-day actuality of living with one.

Thus, we were open and honest with Emily and Daniel about Andrew's illness and expected death. It is a delicate thing, gently introducing children to the concept of death, and especially to its permanence. It is even more delicate to explain the permanence of death while encouraging a relationship with the sibling destined to be taken away. There were tears, and certainly there were questions impossible to answer, such as "Why?" Yet our family carried on. Emily and Daniel did not withdraw or behave outrageously to themselves or others. Among our treasured photos are pictures of Emily and Daniel holding their brother outside the ICU. He was still attached to intravenous lines and bandaged and hung limply in their arms, but his siblings are smiling proudly while helping out with a brother, as any other family member would.

Now, years later, both children have accepted Andrew's severe disability and his unusual physical dependence on them. His special needs are matter-of-factly accommodated but do not consume the course of the day. Given Andrew's weakness and inability to move himself or most objects more than a short distance, it is perhaps unavoidable that Ruth and I have relied on Emily and Daniel to help with physically lifting Andrew and bringing his environment to him. I continue to be amazed at their simple acceptance of demanding duties that most adults, much less all their peers, have never had to consider performing.

It has always been my opinion, however, that the real value of Andrew's siblings must lie in their ability to bring a *normal childhood* closer to him. A service dog, or a parent with a strong back, can lift and move. There is no substitute, though, for a brother playing tag, or pretending to lose a race, or lobbing very soft pitches meant to be hit by even the weakest of swings. The intangible benefits of a sister skating around the neighborhood with Andrew on a warm spring day far outweigh the brief help that having her lift her brother on and off the toilet would offer to us. Emily and Daniel are first and foremost children, not therapists. I believe that regarding his siblings as siblings, not as therapists or aids, will continue to maintain a healthy relationship between all three. Just as importantly, such an attitude will hopefully help Andrew simply be a child.

Ruth and I are careful not to keep the realities of Andrew's condition hidden. Our paranoia and the reality of serious relapse are not covered up, which may even bring us all a little closer. So far, all three children remain happy and involved with the natural activities and concerns of childhood. Such a course may have happened anyway simply on the basis of Andrew's gradual improvement, but I can't help but feel the guidance and openness early on helped shape their well-adjusted natures of the present day.

Our strategy of honest confrontation was not based on advice from mental health professionals. We did, however, seek help from child psychologists and social workers throughout the crisis. Despite my admitted distrust, the entire family benefited from the guidance of the professionals we spoke to. For some families, advice from professional outsiders regarding childrearing may be resented or simply ignored. We accepted the fact that keeping a family healthy through the reality of a terminally ill baby was a truly overwhelming task and deserved all the reliable help we could muster. Emily continued to receive counseling from a child psychologist for years. I would unequivocally recommend such intervention for family members of any age forced to cope with situations such as ours.

One other important aspect of sibling care deserves mention. A child who requires constant or special attention to serious illness or basic needs may consume a substantial amount of a parent's time and energy. To a certain degree, this is unavoidable. We have witnessed, however, how sometimes attention to the healthy siblings can be neglected. It may be done unconsciously, in the name of attending to the more obvious and tangible needs of the special needs sibling. But a healthy family depends on the health and inclusion of all members. It is admittedly impossible to devote equal time and attention; the unaffected siblings, after all, aren't equal. Neither, however, can normal childhood concerns be shortchanged. It is yet another delicate balance that is arrived at through individual experience and a certain degree of sensitivity to seemingly trivial concerns that may not be all that trivial when accumulated over years. Those concerns may understandably be at times overlooked, but they must not be forever ignored.

My experiences are not meant to demonstrate an absolute right or wrong way to connect children with adult issues of disability and death. Although a clear cause-and-effect relationship can't be assured, I can say that our family's health up to the current time is a source of great comfort. The strength that comes from healthy relationships among parents and children and among sick and healthy siblings provides a considerable cushion against the daily turmoil of a child's illness. I attribute our family stability to the approach and philosophy I have described, and I feel it offers a helpful model for others confronting similar obstacles.

Respite and Hospice Care

Convincing well-meaning outsiders that a baby's or child's interests are best served only by maintaining comfort in the face of terminal illness can be a surprisingly difficult endeavor for parents. Simply caressing or hugging an infant when serious problems arise instead of calling 911 or rushing the child to an emergency room is extremely uncomfortable for most people to even consider. In my experience, explaining one's actions can be more trying than actually making the decision. Relatives and friends may feel that such a course of action is equivalent to giving up on a child.

Parents must always remain aware that no matter how well-meaning the intentions of friends or family members may be, they can't understand all that goes into making decisions for the critically or terminally ill child. Nor can most understand that the resolve to provide only comfort is as active, as intensive, and as taxing an intervention as would be confronting unknown or serious problems for any child. It is not "doing nothing"; it is exercising restraint under conditions in which the natural reaction is to demand that everything be done. We were disappointed when even home care professionals found our wishes difficult to understand, much less comply with.

My wife and I subsequently sought out hospice care for Andrew, as we were determined to have him live with us at home—and die with us at home. Hospice organizations are designed to allow terminally ill people to die at home, with dignity and in comfort. Nurses, physicians, clergy, and social workers do everything possible to assure that such patients can remain at home despite advanced illness. Pain is managed with supervised narcotics. Shortness of breath and other physical discomforts are treated with appropriate medications and emotional support. Family members are assisted with whatever terminal care is required to allow their loved one to remain comfortable. When the inevitable occurs, a hospice contact person is appropriately called, so that ambulances, emergent trips to the hospital, and futile resuscitative measures are avoided. Hospice is not designed to provide round-the-clock nursing care, but only to assist the family with medical and emotional needs, so they may provide adequate care for a terminal relative. Hospice services are usually paid for by standard health insurance plans, as long as a physician is able to confirm a terminal illness and limited life expectancy. In general a life expectancy of six months or less is felt to warrant hospice care, but in my experience there is obviously a certain amount of uncertainty permitted.

The members of the hospice organization we contacted were kind and understanding and provided appropriately compassionate people to help us with Andrew's needs. Incredibly, no hospice organization in our state had ever taken on the responsibility for a terminal patient as young as Andrew, which was initially even more unsettling for us. Either infants such as Andrew had not survived long enough to make home care a consideration, or other parents caught up in our circumstances had not felt comfort care for a child was appropriate. Given the misconceptions shared by many people never personally or professionally involved with such issues, I suspect it was because of the latter. In any case, the hospice team members pitched in selflessly, willing to help and learn without focusing on possible legal or contractual implications. For parents coping with this uncommon situation, I would definitely advise investigating what the local hospice organization could offer, regardless of social stigma, family or physician pressure, or insurance coverage.

Unfortunately, the hospice organization was not allowed to provide all our necessary home care, causing us to seek help from standard home care providers again. We called several more associations, offering to release them in writing from any duties other than providing simple respite care for us and comfort for Andrew. Today, respite care is typically offered by home health associations and some state Medicaid or Medicare programs. It is designed to provide temporary home care for sick children, children with disabilities, or their relatives. Parents or other caregivers can thus be relieved of responsibility for short but merciful periods of time, allowing them to enjoy other activities or simply to rest. In contrast to hospice care, respite care is not necessarily designed to assist with assuring a comfortable and dignified death for terminal patients. Respite care can be provided by trained or untrained people, and is designed to relieve family members for short periods of time. Providers tend to basic needs of sick or terminally ill patients while they are at home, but do not typically have the sophistication or training to supervise medications or other aspects of terminal care. They should, however, be able to respect wishes for terminal care without interfering.

After repeated rejections, we gave up on obtaining help outside of hospice and family. Perhaps we were naïve in believing that organizations trained to administer home care could liberalize their duties to include comfort care of a child, as long as such care would be helpful *and* reimbursed. We found that the finality of allowing a comfortable death for a child is apparently too much for home care, as opposed to hospice care, professionals to undertake. This situation is perhaps made somewhat more understandable by the prevalence of legal recourse and recriminations in the medical field.

Parents need to be aware of the professional organizations available to provide emotional and medical support in the home. Moreover, they need to be aware of the merits and obstacles involved in bringing more health care professionals into a personal and difficult situation. In the extreme circumstance of caring for a child with devastating disabilities or terminal illness, hospice care may be the only outlet for unconditional support and respite. If our experience can be generalized, however, it appears as if many hospice workers have rarely, if ever, been approached by a pediatrician or the parents of a very young patient. Furthermore, hospice care hours tend to be limited. Home care nursing associations may not be permitted to take up the slack.

One unexpected aspect of hospice care deserves to be mentioned. Several of the hospice workers who helped out in homes such as ours turned out to be survivors of their own personal family tragedies. The caregiver who was assigned to Andrew had herself lost a child to cancer years before. She provided the physical in-home presence we needed while respecting the limits of care we requested. In time, she provided a compassionate outlet for our frustrations and feelings, and she eventually became a trusted friend as well as a hired hospice worker. It probably shouldn't have come as such a surprise that some of these survivors would want to put their experiences to use for others. Perhaps the surprise really lay in how such simple empathy and unreserved compassion could be obtained from a health care provider organization as dependent on matters of reimbursement and regulated referral as any other modern health care provider. Many associations offering hospice care may harbor such unpublicized and untapped sources of emotional support.

Chapter 4

The Child with a Disability

We had repeatedly been assured by pediatricians, pediatric intensivists, and renowned neurologists that within several years of his birth, Andrew would no longer be with us. Now, years later, we still have three children, not two. Andrew remains physically disabled, but he is alive and has a future that was previously thought to be impossible. He somehow avoided requiring life support when overwhelmed by the RSV pneumonia, then made it home against the odds. Predicted to finally succumb when the feeding tube was removed, Andrew made all the discussions and preparations for his death moot. He became one of the only children in our state to be deemed appropriate for and to be placed into hospice care. He then became one of only a few people who outlived "terminal" and actually graduated from hospice care.

Andrew has thus defeated the odds many times over by living and thriving years longer than the doomed infancy the best specialists had predicted. Today he is alive, seven years old, happy, and thriving. Any one of these descriptions would have been impossible to apply to Andrew at the beginning. That all four terms now describe our son is nothing short of miraculous. He remains extremely weak, unable to sit up, roll over, or move himself more than a few inches. The development of any cough at all becomes a source of unimaginable anxiety for his parents. Even today, images of what so many patients suffer through with respiratory infections are conjured up by the sound of a simple cough. Andrew, however, remains oblivious, virtually ignoring the colds that torture his parents who have seen and who know too much.

He is in command of a 150 pound power wheelchair, and maneuvers it deftly both inside and outside. He is completing first grade in a public school where teachers and para-professionals could not be more supportive and compassionate. It is an optimistic childhood so far, but never free from glaring reminders of disability. His classmates are carpooled to and from soccer games, baseball games, dance lessons, and judo after school; physical therapy, aquatic therapy, occupational therapy, and doctor appointments are Andrew's after-school activities. His friends dress themselves for school each day with little thought; Ruth virtually girds Andrew for battle each morning in his stiff body jacket, ankle braces, and mechanized wheelchair. Through it all, Andrew remains, still, a seven-year-old kid, with seven-year-old enthusiasm. It has been a journey mysterious enough to defeat anyone's ability to determine what's going to happen.

Is it fair to call all this miraculous? All we know is that these aspects of Andrew's life haven't been explained or predicted yet. I do know that watching Andrew live against the odds with his illness has allowed me to believe in at least the possibility of unlikely outcomes for patients. I can tell patients what to realistically expect out of a serious illness on the basis of science and fact. I can also, with sincerity and credibility, leave room to hope for an unlikely outcome. I would never encourage unrealistic expectations, but I would not destroy hope either. Whether miracles happen or whether medical science simply has not progressed far enough to allow a rational explanation of everything that happens to patients is a matter of speculation. I prefer to dwell on the certainty of at least some small hope in every situation and leave explanations to those who have the luxury to spend time on such musings.

I have also come to realize that a child should be allowed to be a kid, regardless of whatever medical turmoil swirls about them. When illness or disability intrudes, *child* and *kid* become different things. In the face of childhood disability, doctor appointments, therapies, and rigorous efforts toward healing may become the focus. A *child* endures these treatments and grows up far too quickly. A *kid* simply wants to get started with Nintendo or go swinging outside. Whether a child is terminally ill or chronically disabled, being a kid may be among the most therapeutic treatments of all. In my experience, helping a child be a kid despite hardship can also be amazingly therapeutic for a parent.

I have chosen to dedicate myself to finding ways of making a severely physically challenged child feel like any other child and helping him enjoy life as much as possible. I rely on the input of the professionals we have assembled—the physicians, specialists, and therapists—to make sure Andrew, as a child with a disability, is not deprived of any new developments or treatments. I feel, however, that with other neighborhood children running around and enjoying the sunshine, Andrew the kid would benefit more if I found interesting outdoor sights instead of seeking interesting Websites. I have known parents who combated helplessness in the face of a child's illness by perusing the Internet and constantly pursuing options, opinions, and more facts about disease and treatments. It is a parent's responsibility to try to achieve a balance between researching therapies for a child with a disability and ensuring childhood enjoyment for a kid. Certainly they are not mutually exclusive endeavors. I have chosen the pursuit of childhood activities.

So we greet each lost tooth with a concerted effort to contact the Tooth Fairy. We play football in the fall, although it's more enjoyable for Andrew to actually *be* the football instead of playing football (the pitch-outs are breathtaking). We wrestle at night, an activity in which Andrew becomes a physical giant. Outdoor swings provide the sensation of movement and rushing wind that an otherwise immobile kid would have difficulty creating and allows time in the sun. They are all weapons against the despondency that chronic illness can so easily inflict by shoving normal childhood into a harsher reality. The physical therapy, the doctor's visits, and the medical literature are not ignored or neglected. We just need distraction from them.

If I could express thanks for whatever miracle or whatever unknown medical process that has bestowed upon my son a longer childhood, simply celebrating that childhood while he lives it seems as genuine and as healing a way to do it as any.

Membership in "The Club"

There are all sorts of exclusive clubs to join. Most have memberships that are greedily coveted. Membership in other clubs, however, is thrust upon reluctant innocents. One such club is exclusively open to parents of children with disabilities. The Club is not a support group for people who share common concerns. The Club is a shared state of disconnection forced upon parents. Different perspectives and life experiences don't necessarily drive parents apart; the refusal or inability to understand and respect different perspectives does. The exclusivity that members share is based on the tangible and obvious requirement of raising a child who has disabilities. But the exclusivity is also the result of the lack of insight and consideration that many nonmembers demonstrate. Although rarely malicious or purposeful, such apparent insensitivity sets members of The Club apart as surely as physical segregation does. We have had friends complain to us how their seven-month-old just wasn't walking as well as all the other children they knew. At the time, we were trying to prop up our own seven-month-old, who had no muscle tone at all, couldn't roll over by himself, and was expected to die prematurely. Other parents, some good friends, other casual acquaintances, have poured out their troubles to us about pigeon-toed sons, picky eaters, and late toilet trainers. They are not simply commenting; they are complaining to us. And we have seen friends park in reserved handicapped parking spaces so as to permit themselves and their children—all perfectly capable of walking—as little inconvenience as possible.

The list could go on, but these brief examples should suffice to illustrate what drives membership in The Club. Each example is trivial and doesn't even merit a second thought from those parents or family friends. Each experience, in isolation, is even an understandable concern or action for the usual parent absorbed in usual childhood concerns (except taking advantage of reserved parking). After all, what parents wouldn't want the best for their child? What parents wouldn't be concerned over their child's milestones and development? No, it is not the actual words and comments that are so damaging.

Damage is done through oblivious self-absorption and total disregard of the need for such normal concerns to be put in the proper perspective when faced with others caught up in more extraordinary circumstances. Few parents of children with disabilities would ask that special accommodations or actions be observed in order to equalize conditions or share misery. Few would wish their daily responsibilities or burdens on others. For most, it is not a question of revenge to somehow exact on those who have not yet been visited by unexpected hardship. Parents in The Club do not obtain comfort from expressions of pity or gushing utterances of sympathy. Steadfastly ignoring the glaring reality of a mentally or physically challenged child and carrying on as if a wheelchair or disability didn't exist at all usually offers little comfort either. Isolation in The Club becomes less likely to occur only when otherwise normal anxieties and issues are not accorded inappropriate importance when confronted by more weighty concerns. This opinion is not meant to represent the perspective held by all parents who share my circumstances. It is based on Ruth's and my experiences, as well as on opinions gathered from other parents Ruth and I talked with during our children's therapy sessions, while waiting at a school for disabled children, and during support group discussions.

Unfortunately, members of the medical community are often just as guilty of unintentional insensitivity. Certainly a shooting-the-messenger response from distraught parents can be expected. My own experience with physicians has run the gamut from extraordinary compassion under the most trying of circumstances for all involved to painful business-as-usual insensitivity. These words are not written lightly, therefore, or without the sincerest attempt to maintain responsible objectivity. As previous chapters have related, Ruth and I will always remember and treasure the truly compassionate physicians who supported us through our darkest times. Since I have spent time on the other side of medical care and have spoken with parents in the same position as I am, I can also attest, however, that the insensitive words and hurtful interactions linger and fester even more vividly than the positive moments. I have been astounded at how blatantly insensitive physicians can be in situations requiring the most delicate of interactions. Strangely, many such instances have occurred among the very health care professionals who deal almost daily with the most tragic of childhood illnesses.

"What can we expect him to eventually do?" one mother asked of a pediatric neurologist about her son, who had a rare structural brain abnormality.

"I wouldn't worry too much," the neurologist responded almost condescendingly. "He'll probably be able to at least pay taxes one day."

Another mother told us of a conversation regarding her daughter who was afflicted with a rare chromosomal disorder called *cri-du-chat* (literally, "cry of the cat" in French, named after the peculiar high-pitched wail affected children display). Voicing her anxiety over her child's future potential, she was cautioned by her pediatric neurologist against too much concern. "After all," he went on to add, "By the time she's thirteen, she'll be sitting in a corner chewing on an old shoe."

An objective observer could make the observation that for every such example, two or three examples of very compassionate interaction and care exist among physicians. This may very well be true. Indeed, our own most grateful memories of physician support have been accorded due respect in this book. But the damage wreaked by a pitiless attitude or by a remark so insensitive as to steal hope can undo all previous kindness and forever generate suspicion and defensiveness.

Our own experiences with the medical establishment from the other side have permanently changed our lives as physicians as well as our attitudes as parents. Since Andrew's birth, Ruth has not returned to work. The majority of pediatric practice involves care of the healthy child and attention to normal developmental progress. Ruth has been simply unable to accord the proper consideration to such issues when confronted with issues of life and death, chronic disability, and neuromuscular disease at home. Moreover, as a pediatrician Ruth was expected to follow a pediatric patient's normal development and offer assurance with each developmental milestone that a child achieved. As the mother of a severely developmentally delayed child, Ruth quickly became emotionally devastated by such a responsibility, and could barely keep from taking out her frustration on undeserving parents.

Our move from Rhode Island to Kansas was prompted by my own inability to tolerate academic medicine after our experiences with Andrew. Using actual patients to teach the practice of medicine, regarding patients as useful subjects for clinical investigations, became increasingly intolerable. When my discomfort turned to barely concealed rage during rounds in the intensive care unit, I knew I could no longer uphold my responsibilities as an academic physician. I couldn't get past memories of large groups of residents and students descending on my own son's incubator, nor could I block out the entire ordeal of our trip to Boston. I resigned from academic medicine and moved into a private practice position in the Midwest, where reimbursement and private practice opportunities were more plentiful. To this day I actually dread even the small amount of bedside teaching I am required to do as part of my current responsibilities, and still harbor unreasonable resentment towards the students and residents who are only trying to learn by my example.

Parents of seriously ill children or children with disabilities will inevitably feel out of step with the rest of the world. They are pushed into The Club when feeling out of step turns into feeling isolated, overwhelmed, and misunderstood. Health care providers must be aware that flippant words or unthinking impressions can have unintended effects among parents with heightened sensitivity and reduced tolerance. Friends and family members need to be aware that they can rejoice in their own children's health and accomplishments but need to respect that others may be coping with a lack of such fulfillment. Sensitivity shouldn't have to be that difficult; people shouldn't have to experience their own tragedies to appreciate another parent's pain, any more than walking through coals isn't necessary to realize how much a burn hurts. In our experience, though, self-absorption all too often trumps empathy.

On the other hand, members of The Club need to remain aware that others simply can't know exactly what they experience every day. It's unfortunately easy, and even therapeutic in the short run, to lash out at unsuspecting acquaintances who get in the way of frustration. The wounds can linger long after the therapeutic benefits fade, and can drive people further into The Club's isolation. Only efforts at awareness on the part of members and nonmembers alike can start to whittle down the membership into this fraternity of frustration.

Dot-Com Caution

As we have become more involved with various rehabilitative organizations, my wife and I have been struck by three realizations. First, there are an amazing number of rehabilitative specialists and innovative appliances that have become available to help children with all types of disabilities. Second, there are an amazing number of families who have no idea that those resources are available. Many don't have the technological sophistication or knowledge to even know where or how to begin to investigate such resources. They are then left to tolerate their child's disability instead of obtaining help that may help reduce disability. Internet accessibility and specialty magazines on relevant topics have helped such families. They have opened up to parents a major weapon in their fight against adversity: knowledge. In fact, the Internet has revolutionized communication about disability in the same way as assisted technology has revolutionized the treatment of disability. Parents can very easily find themselves overwhelmed and faced with either too little or too much information to allow any real progress.

The third realization that struck us follows directly from this last consideration. Many parents still carry on day to day without the help of these resources, or they rely on rudimentary do-it-yourself home rehabilitation. They trudge their way through each day despite all this Internet accessibility and ready information. One reason may be the ever-increasing amount of information itself. Websites, journals, and cybertherapies can easily build up into an avalanche that can overwhelm and bury parents instead of guide them. Recommendations and guidance from distant sources are simply words. All the Website wisdom and dot-com camaraderie in the world won't substitute for the living person who can sort through the avalanche of information, determine what's reliable and helpful, and then put words into action. Dot-com glamour gets all the press. In many cases, however, disability is battled down in the trenches, with therapists and specialists willing to devote hands-on treatment and assume responsibility for advice and guidance. Websites won't stretch out contractures, instruct the proper way to transfer without injuring backs or joints, or individualize computer learning for mentally challenged children.

These words of caution haven't arisen from unreasonable intimidation of computers or technology. Andrew has benefited from technology; his power wheelchair and e-mail communication have opened up his world more than would even have been imagined if he had been born decades earlier. Nonetheless, even given our medical knowledge, we have relied heavily on the advice of physical therapists and pediatric rehabilitative specialists to sort through all the options. We certainly have depended on flesh-and-blood resources over electrons to work directly with Andrew and slow the relentless physical effects of neuromuscular weakness.

Words of caution come from experience with patients as well. Many times patients have come into my office clutching the latest development gleaned from the Internet. The optimism they radiate is often refreshing, perhaps because they feel that for the first time since receiving their diagnosis, they have gained some sense of control over it. Many times, however, the news or information they bring to me has only a key word in common with their actual circumstances. The Internet can be a map or a maze, depending on the guidance available to help negotiate it. It is rare that information or a discovery vital to a patient's recovery can be culled from the Internet without appearing in medical literature as well, and physicians keep abreast of medical literature.

Certainly the Internet offers an incredible opportunity to generate unity and support among parents coping with children with disabilities. Communication between families miles away can inspire hope and optimism, can occasionally uncover new ideas or options, and unquestionably can open up the world to children otherwise limited by their conditions. I don't take lightly the good fortune of our in-home elevator, our ramp-equipped van, Andrew's power wheelchair, or our desktop and laptop computers. Andrew has become more electronically empowered than was imagined in my own childhood.

The balanced perspective of our reliance on technology, therefore, lends more credibility to the precautions voiced in this chapter. The value of moving into the previously unimaginable future of mouse-driven magic and joystick mastery should not totally overshadow the more pedestrian but therapeutic benefits of human contact and personalized help.

Therapy People

Obtaining the appropriate rehabilitative services for a child with a disability is one situation where a parent's persistence, even insistence, can make a huge difference. Complicated diagnostic evaluations, sophisticated tests, and medications are all the responsibilities of the pediatrician or specialist. Progress achieved through slower, more tedious, less glorified interventions on the part of other health care professionals may become even more important over the long run for many children with disabilities, but they may not be readily prescribed. Many physicians may have inadequate knowledge of all the options available for rehabilitation, mainly out of a lack of experience with children with disabilities. Interestingly, some of the most insightful suggestions and observations regarding Andrew's care and progress have come from involved physical therapists, occupational therapists, speech pathologists, and appliance specialists. Andrew's paraprofessional at school, who has no medical training, has contributed invaluable assessments and ideas no one had ever before considered.

Why should this revelation come as such a surprise? These professionals often spend hours with children instead of relying on a twenty- or thirty-minute office visit to formulate an impression. They have the opportunity to observe children in settings where their abilities and disabilities can be viewed naturally, instead of watching them in an artificial and momentary setting of the physician office examining table. These specialists are allowed to watch incremental progress over days, weeks, and months, and can adjust what they do according to both the short-term and long-term changes they observe. Andrew refers to these professionals as his "Therapy People." We have come to rely on all his Therapy People not only for the professional interventions they are trained to administer but also for their innovative ideas and observations. They have become *our* Therapy People.

I cannot offer a comprehensive list of all the possible resources available to parents. Appropriate resources will depend on each child's individual illness or disability. Many electronic and print sources can offer parents general and specific information on particular disabilities. The National Information Center for Children and Youth with Disabilities (www.nichcy.org) provides lists of resources for almost every disability or illness a parent could seek help for. And the magazine *Exceptional Parent* offers a list of resources every year for many disabilities and illnesses. For the child with severe physical disability such as Andrew's, specific resources include aquatic therapy, standard land-based physical therapy, occupational therapy, and horseback-riding therapy. The input from wheelchair seating specialists and orthotists (specialists in prosthetics and braces) has also proven valuable. Andrew's school district offers technology and computer specialists as well as an adaptive physical education teacher. And as mentioned above, the paraprofessional at Andrew's school is truly invested in his welfare and has provided insights into how Andrew copes, what activities and therapies are beneficial or useless, and what innovations can help him handle his environment.

Centers that combine such services into an integrated staff seem to work most smoothly and reduce complexity in parents' already complicated lives. Independent therapists are no less able to make a difference in a child's life, however. They simply need to take their responsibilities seriously enough and to realize how important a role they can have. Parents need to realize these services and resources are available. Pediatricians, children's hospitals, and rehabilitation centers can all offer a reasonable starting point to direct parents to appropriate therapy. Parents also need to accept that the unglamorous and often underestimated professionals in the health care system offer not only specific occupational and physical therapy, but also emotional support, intelligent observations, and intuitive guidance through extended interactions.

These professionals rarely effect dramatic or sudden improvement by their repetitious therapies. Of course, the reality for most physically challenged or cognitively challenged children is not Hollywood-style moments of sudden improvements or inspired cures. There always remains cause for hope, and improvement can indeed occur. Our experience certainly demonstrates that. But it usually comes as the result of tedious daily determination and devoted patience. The bottom line is that living with a child with a disability is often a team effort, a team that involves parents and other family members, physicians, therapists, and teachers. Advice from each member may come from different perspectives and radically different roles within the health care system. It is exactly these differences that make it important not to overlook how important a contribution each individual team member can make to a child's welfare—and to a parent's peace of mind.

Chapter 5

Final Perspectives

Confronting any serious illness and the ravages it may inflict such as chronic disability, physical discomfort, financial hardship, or terminal outlook should be regarded as nothing less than fighting a war. The enemy itself may be invisible, hidden within weakened muscles, malfunctioning brain cells, plugged bronchial tubes, or cancerous organs. The prisoners it takes, however, are all too evident and all too real.

Just as in actual war, the war against childhood illness is fought in the long run, with each individual battle or skirmish making a difference. For both my patients and my own son, victory is rarely achieved by attaining overwhelming conquest of illness or by vanquishing medical concerns in total. Victory is declared with very small gains, especially when the enemy poses such dishearteningly insurmountable obstacles daily. Some parents can declare victory in the war simply by getting out of bed in the morning and refusing to surrender hope. Andrew seizes a decisive victory in one small battle by rolling over one day by himself after years of frustration.

A patient of mine with amyotrophic lateral sclerosis (ALS) wishes desperately for a cure to be found so that one day she will get out of her wheelchair and walk. This is from a woman who has become totally paralyzed and can't breathe without a ventilator. I want to assure her that she has already conquered her disease. Even if she never moved a muscle again, she has risen above anything ALS could do to her by keeping her faith, by continuing to nurture her love of music and other hobbies, and by teaching the rest of us what true strength really is.

Likewise, there are parents every day who get up, lift their child from bed to wheelchair, feed their child through a tube instead of with utensils, and carry on with life. Victories of the spirit count as much in battle as anything else. That is not to say that more dramatic victories aren't extremely uplifting: news of a negative X-ray film after years of chemotherapy; pneumonia cured despite weakened breathing muscles; successful treatment of a tumor considered incurable. At such times, children and parents alike fire a virtual broadside against the enemy and are able to carry on, inspired, into the next battle.

Overly dramatic? Not to the people who fight the battles daily and who never have the luxury of assuming they'll eventually emerge victorious. As a pulmonary physician, I frequently see patients who can no longer see the light at the end of the tunnel as they confront lung cancer or end-stage emphysema. Sometimes all that can be said are words of honest recognition of the small but meaningful victories they have achieved in their own personal war. As the parent of a child whose every independent movement is a triumph, I can appreciate the significance of small victories in each personal war against adversity. Sometimes, though, I wish I could rotate off the front lines for a while.

Final Answers—or Just More Questions?

Occasionally in medicine events occur that appear on the surface to be nothing short of miraculous. Such unexpected outcomes are typically explained as examples of the fallibility of medical science even in this age of sophisticated tests and technological breakthroughs. Our previously terminally ill child exemplifies the miracles in and the frailty of modern medicine, as Andrew remains not only alive but thriving far beyond what was predicted. Our optimism must be tempered by the still variable prognosis of his illness, but *unknown* definitely beats *invariably fatal.* Does this turn of events, however, cast all our previous decisions in a more suspect light? Decisions made out of love and made on the basis of what we considered to be our child's best interests? After all, we had refused to prolong our child's life through painful and uncomfortable interventions that would not have altered his terminal prognosis anyway—a prognosis that was eventually proven wrong.

Does this scenario invalidate all the objective opinions and statements promulgated in this book? Had Ruth and I fallen into a trap discussed in the articles previously mentioned: "Health care professionals should not use their judgment of the patient's quality of life to justify withholding life-sustaining therapy." (*American Journal of Physical Medicine & Rehabilitation*, 1991 June 70:129)? These studies looked only at adults, not infants or children. We had to make decisions for an infant *unable to even understand* what was being done for him, much less share in the decision. Furthermore, we were acting in the capacity of parents destined to live the daily repercussions of that decision, not as health care professionals responsible only to guide and support from a professional distance.

These articles, therefore, are not relevant to all such ethical situations, especially those situations in which children are involved. They do provide a valuable beginning to guide the medical profession through these issues. I included them in this book because they represent admirable attempts to place intangible, subjective, and previously neglected values and issues into a scientific peer-reviewed process. Certainly these dilemmas have always been very real for the families confronting them personally. Confronting them through the objectivity of medical literature provides the credibility and frame of reference upon which the medical community's involvement can be enhanced. This hopefully will lead to more understanding among health care professionals.

On a larger scale, do my family's experiences really prove that everything should always be done to preserve a child's life regardless of the predicted prognosis, the anticipated quality of life, or the extent of measures required to sustain his or her life? Andrew has certainly illustrated that the best of educated medical pronouncements regarding prognosis could be proven wrong. The emotions and controversies surrounding a very ill child deserve the difficult nature of these questions.

I can look back over everything that has happened to us without regretting the decisions Ruth and I made and the actions we took. Our decisions were made out of the utmost concern for our child's welfare and were the very best we could do as parents under those demoralizing conditions. We acted on the only information we had at the time: information that was based on the opinions of multiple specialists and redundant sophisticated testing—essentially on everything that modern medicine could offer to help guide us through the turmoil of serious childhood illness.

We could have acted on a dogmatic view of a future in which anything was possible given enough hope and faith. Illness could somehow get better, no matter what the tests or doctors say, so do everything in preparation for that. To do anything less, to prepare to succumb in peace, would be to simply give up. In our situation, it would have been the right course of action. Andrew did overcome the odds; he did defeat the prognosis. He made for us and for himself a future where no future was expected to exist at all.

We had no crystal ball, however, through which to view the future and plan and act accordingly. Life never works that conveniently for anyone. Parents and other family members responsible for caring for ill children must sometimes make difficult decisions on the basis of personal and individual views on quality of life. A certain course of action or a particular resolve cannot be judged with hindsight and retrospective knowledge of outcome. No one is happier or more thankful than Ruth and I that the outcome we feared was never realized and that the decisions we made never had to be tested. Nor do we regret what we did on Andrew's behalf.

The only certainty we hold now is that so far Andrew has been spared discomfort, and his quality of life has been preserved. Amazingly, his quantity of life is catching up with his quality of life. Our journey with Andrew has led us to see that optimism and hope can still arise out of the worst of circumstances. We have little room now for either regrets or for the need to seek explanations. We have enough trouble just catching up on simple enjoyment.

Printed in the United States
50776LVS00003B/201

9 780595 133079